You Can
Be Happy

You Can
Be Happy

The scientifically proven way to change how you feel

PROFESSOR DANIEL FREEMAN
&
JASON FREEMAN

PEARSON

Harlow, England • London • New York • Boston • San Francisco • Toronto • Sydney
Auckland • Singapore • Hong Kong • Tokyo • Seoul • Taipei • New Delhi
Cape Town • São Paulo • Mexico City • Madrid • Amsterdam • Munich • Paris • Milan

PEARSON EDUCATION LIMITED

Edinburgh Gate
Harlow CM20 2JE
Tel: +44 (0)1279 623623
Fax: +44 (0)1279 431059
Website: www.pearsoned.co.uk

First published in Great Britain in 2012

ISBN: 978-0-273-76390-1

British Library Cataloguing-in-Publication Data
A catalogue record for this book is available from the British Library

Library of Congress Cataloging-in-Publication Data
Freeman, Daniel, 1971-
  You can be happy : the scientifically proven way to change how to feel / Daniel
Freemann & Jason Freeman.
    p. cm.
Includes index.
ISBN 978-0-273-76390-1 (pbk.)
1. Happiness. I. Freeman, Jason (Jason Ryan) II. Title.
  BF575.H27F735 2012
  152.4'2--dc23
                          2011043057

10 9 8 7 6 5 4 3 2 1
16 15 14 13 12

Typeset in 8.5 Sabon by 30
Printed and bound in Great Britain by Clays Ltd., Bungay, Suffolk

Table of contents

About the authors vii
Acknowledgements ix
Publisher's acknowledgements xi
Preface xiii

CHAPTER 1: INTRODUCTION 1

CHAPTER 2: COMMITTING TO HAPPINESS 15

CHAPTER 3: GETTING THE BASICS IN PLACE: IMPROVING YOUR DIET AND SLEEP 25

CHAPTER 4: ACTIVITIES FOR HAPPINESS 37

CHAPTER 5: CALMING NEGATIVE THOUGHTS 55

CHAPTER 6: INCREASING POSITIVE THOUGHTS 69

CHAPTER 7: RELAXING YOUR BODY AND MIND 85

CHAPTER 8: IMPROVING YOUR RELATIONSHIPS 97

CHAPTER 9: HAPPINESS AT WORK 117

CHAPTER 10: UNDERLYING PROBLEMS:
COMMON PSYCHOLOGICAL ISSUES THAT FUEL
UNHAPPINESS 131

CHAPTER 11: BECOMING HAPPIER – AND STAYING
HAPPIER 147

Further reading 157

About the authors

Daniel Freeman is one of the UK's leading clinical psychologists. He is a Professor of Clinical Psychology, a Medical Research Council (MRC) Senior Clinical Fellow and a British Psychological Society Fellow in the Department of Psychiatry at Oxford University.

Jason Freeman is a writer and editor in the areas of popular psychology and self-help.

Daniel and Jason are the authors of several psychology titles, including *Use Your Head: A Guided Tour of the Human Mind* (2010). Their work has appeared in various national newspapers and magazines, among them *The Times*, *The Guardian*, *The Independent* and *Psychologies*.

Acknowledgements

We are extremely grateful to Rachael Stock, our excellent editor at Pearson. *You Can Be Happy* wouldn't be the book it is without her enthusiasm, encouragement and consistently judicious advice.

Many thanks, as ever, to our wonderful agent Zoe King at the Blair Partnership; to the new Oxford psychologists Nicole Butcher and Rachel Lister for their careful reading of the typescript and helpful comments; and to the many friends and family members with whom we've discussed the issues in this book over recent months. With respect to the latter, Daniel would particularly like to acknowledge the birthday dinner discussion with Nick, Mary, Jill and Tom.

One of the key findings of research into happiness is that few things in life are more important for our well-being than the people closest to us. So with this in mind, Jason would like to thank Eleanor, Ethan, Evelyn and Jude: theory in practice!

We are grateful to the authors of the self-assessment questionnaires for permission to include their work in *You Can Be Happy*. The Warwick–Edinburgh Mental Well-being Scale, reproduced on p.11, was funded by the Scottish Executive National Programme for improving mental health and well-being, commissioned by NHS Health Scotland, developed by the University of Warwick and the University of Edinburgh, and is jointly owned by NHS Health Scotland, the University of Warwick and the University of Edinburgh. Web link: http://www.healthscotland.com/understanding/population/Measuring-positive-mental-health.aspx

Publisher's acknowledgements

We are grateful to the following for permission to reproduce copyright material:

The Warwick-Edinburgh Mental Well-being Scale (WEMWBS) on pp.11–12 © NHS Health Scotland, University of Warwick and University of Edinburgh, 2006, all rights reserved; sleep questionnaire on pp.32–3 from Spoormaker, V. I., van den Bout, J., and Klip, E. C., 'Initial validation of the SLEEP-50 questionnaire', *Behavioural Sleep Medicine*, 3, 227–46 (2005) © Taylor & Francis Group (http://www.informaworld.com); VIA Survey on pp.44–5 from Peterson, P. and Seligman, M., *Character Strengths and Virtues: A Handbook Classifcation* (OUP USA, 2004), Copyright 2004 VIA Institute on Character (www.viacharacter.org); Penn State Worry Questionnaire on p.134 from Meyer, T. J., Miller, M. L., Metzger, R. L. and Borkovec, T. D., 'Development and validation of the Penn State Worry Questionnaire', *Behavioural Research and Therapy*, 28, 487–95 (Elsevier, 1990).

In some instances we have been unable to trace the owners of copyright material, and we would appreciate any information that would enable us to do so.

Preface

You Can Be Happy offers something we believe is unique: a concise, accessible and, most importantly, scientifically reliable collection of the practical steps you can take to become happier. The techniques and activities we recommend here have been proven to get results. Make them part of your routine and they will work for you too.

This book is based on the very best psychological research and clinical practice. In particular, it draws on three of the most significant currents in psychology today: Cognitive Behaviour Therapy (CBT), mindfulness and positive psychology.

CBT was first developed in the 1960s by Professor Aaron Beck as a treatment for depression. Since then, it's been used very successfully to help people with many other psychological problems. CBT is based on the insight that if we can understand and change the way we think and the beliefs we hold about ourselves and the world around us, we'll also be able to change the way we feel and behave. Becoming happier involves both calming our negative thoughts and increasing our positive thoughts – objectives CBT is ideally suited to achieve.

Mindfulness is a synthesis of modern Western psychological thinking and ancient Buddhist beliefs and practices, particularly meditation. Mindfulness involves learning to live in the moment, developing your awareness of what it feels like to be alive in this present instant, and understanding that your thoughts and feelings are temporary, transient, and not necessarily a reflection of reality. It's a very effective way of relaxing both mind and body and developing contentment.

Positive psychology was initiated in the late 1990s by the US psychologist Martin Seligman. Arguing that psychology had concentrated too exclusively on mental illness, Seligman called for the study of positive emotions such as happiness. Today positive psychology is thriving, with big advances being made in our understanding of what happiness is and how we can go about increasing it.

These strands of psychological research and clinical practice underpin *You Can Be Happy*. But we've kept the theory and the jargon to an absolute minimum. We think you'll be more interested in what you can actually *do*, here and now, to become happier. And the good news is that you can do a great deal.

With the right guidance, we can all become happier. *You Can Be Happy* will show you how.

CHAPTER 1
Introduction

There are only two ways to live your life. One is as though nothing is a miracle. The other is as though everything is a miracle. ALBERT EINSTEIN

Happiness is far too important to leave to chance. You know that, of course. It's just that life has a habit of getting in the way.

Perhaps things are more stressful or complicated than they used to be. Maybe you feel you've forgotten how to be happy. Or that you're just 'not a happy person'. Perhaps you don't know where the happiness went – or how to get it back.

But whatever your situation, you can take control.

You can learn how to increase your sense of well-being.

You can become happier.

In this book you will discover the very best techniques, based on the most up-to-date science, to calm your negative emotions and to bring happiness towards the centre of your life. These techniques have worked for very many people, and we believe they will work for you too. You really can achieve the change you want so much, step by step and day by day.

WHAT IS HAPPINESS?

We all know happiness when we experience it. We may not consciously think to ourselves: 'I am happy now', but we instinctively recognise and relish its presence. And when happiness deserts us, we long for its return.

But it pays to spend a moment considering what happiness actually is. If we think about and appreciate the various forms of happiness, we know what it is we're striving for. And the techniques presented in this book will make more sense. Philosophers, scientists and artists have been debating the nature of happiness since at least ancient Greek times, and it's a discussion that is still very much ongoing. There are dozens of interpretations of happiness. Nevertheless, a broad consensus has emerged among psychologists that happiness has three key components:

● Pleasure

● Meaning

● Engagement

And we believe a fourth is implicit in the research findings. It's an aspect that doesn't get much attention in books about happiness, but one we think is just as important as the others:

● Fewer negative emotions

Pleasure

Pleasure is what we're all hard-wired to pursue. It's the elation we feel when our team scores a goal, the delight we experience when we see an old friend again, the wonderful sensation of eating delicious food or tasting superb wine, the contentment that comes with finishing a difficult piece of work.

This *hedonic* type of happiness is all about feeling good in the moment. It's one of the five basic emotions alongside sadness, fear, anger and disgust. By basic, we mean the first to develop in humans, usually within the first six months after birth.

Meaning

Charles M. Schulz, creator of the *Peanuts* comic strip, once wrote: 'My life has no purpose, no direction, no aim, no meaning, and yet I'm happy. I can't figure it out. What am I doing right?' In fact, Schulz reportedly took just one holiday during the entire fifty-year run of *Peanuts*, which suggests his life was full of meaning.

It doesn't matter where you find the meaning in your life: it might be your career, family, hobby, religion or political activism. What matters is that you're looking outwards and *connecting* to something greater than yourself.

Focusing your life solely on making a buck shows a certain poverty of ambition. It asks too little of yourself. Because it's only when you hitch your wagon to something larger than yourself that you realise your true potential. BARACK OBAMA

Engagement

Have you ever been so absorbed in what you were doing that you were oblivious to time, your surroundings, even your own thoughts? Perhaps you were playing a musical instrument, working on a project, cooking, or engrossed in a crossword puzzle. Some people experience the feeling when they're behind a camera. This sense of being so completely focused on the task at hand that you lose all sense of yourself is engagement or *flow*.

I was already on pole ... and I just kept going. Suddenly I was nearly two seconds faster than anybody else, including my team mate with the same car. And suddenly I realised that I was no longer driving the car consciously. I was driving it by a kind of instinct, only I was in a different dimension. It was like I was in a tunnel. AYRTON SENNA

Fewer negative emotions

Unpleasant feelings such as anger, anxiety and depression are inevitable at some point in our life. And they can be useful: anxiety, for example, is designed to warn us of potential danger. But these feelings are so powerful that they can prevent us from experiencing pleasure, meaning and engagement. By reducing the amount of time we spend experiencing negative emotions, we make it possible to enjoy more happiness.

> *By reducing the amount of time we spend experiencing negative emotions, we make it possible to enjoy more happiness.*

The techniques and activities in this book will show you how to improve all four of these aspects of happiness. Luckily the components are connected, so when you tackle one you're likely also to nudge the others along.

How will you know whether you've got it right? You'll notice that your life is increasingly full of what the psychologist Barbara Fredrickson calls the 'ten forms of positivity'. As you read the list, remember the feeling. When did you last feel these emotions? Can you think of a moment when these feelings were especially strong?

- Joy
- Gratitude
- Serenity
- Interest
- Hope
- Pride

- Amusement
- Inspiration
- Awe
- Love

HOW MUCH CONTROL OVER OUR HAPPINESS DO WE REALLY HAVE?

We all have much more influence over our happiness than we often assume. Hence the title of this book!

Everyone can become happier, but our emotions are also influenced by factors over which we often have limited control. Recognising this can be a big help as we try to make sense of our current level of happiness. It also means we shouldn't judge ourselves too harshly if we're not as happy as we'd like to be.

Circumstances

As we all know, life can throw some very big obstacles in our way. Certain situations make happiness tricky to achieve no matter how courageously we pursue it.

For example, illness, bereavement, joblessness, money difficulties, relationship problems and other stressful situations are likely to bring us down, at least for a while. We'd hardly be human if they didn't.

We tend to think of emotions as exclusively personal, but in fact the way we feel is often influenced by what's going on in society as a whole. Difficult economic times, for example, mean increased stress for many.

But social factors can work to increase happiness as well as reduce it. Denmark, for example, is one of the happiest nations on the planet. One of the reasons why Danes are so cheerful is thought to be the country's highly progressive tax system, which ensures that wealth inequality is kept to a minimum.

This matters because we know that one very effective way to make yourself unhappy is to compare yourself to other people. If you fall into the habit, you'll soon discover someone who seems to be doing much better than you. In Denmark, however, a doctor is unlikely to be much more wealthy than, say, a plumber. Consequently, this type of social comparison is far less damaging. It's an ethos nicely encapsulated in the Danish term *Jante-lov*: 'You're no better than anyone else.'

Age

In general, people seem to begin their lives with a high degree of contentment before gradually sliding down the happiness curve. The trickiest time is generally reached in the forties. After this mid-life point, happiness tends to steadily improve. By the time we get to old age, our happiness levels are likely to be pretty much what they were in childhood.

You might be surprised by this turnaround: we live in a culture, after all, that celebrates youth. But the data is very clear: older people are happier than middle-aged folk. (We are, of course, talking averages here: broad statistical trends. Your personal experience may be quite different. A miserable middle age is *not* inevitable!)

Genes

Our personality is partly a result of our genes, and our personality influences our level of happiness.

Two personality traits are especially important: *extraversion* and *neuroticism*. People high in extraversion are pleasure-seekers. They crave thrills, adventure and fun. They are tuned to the positive.

Very neurotic people, on the other hand, are sensitive to the negative in life. To them the world can feel like a minefield, with disaster potentially lurking just around the corner. You won't be surprised to learn that people high in extraversion tend to be happier than people with strong levels of neuroticism.

Our level of happiness, then, is inevitably influenced by our circumstances, our age and by our genes. *Influenced, but not determined.* These factors mean we all tend to start off at different levels of happiness. But regardless of your age, your personality, or your life situation, you can be happier, and we'll show you how.

This isn't to say that these factors are unimportant; far from it. But remember that they are only part of the story. They contribute to your current level of happiness, certainly, but there is plenty of evidence that a *larger* contribution is made by the conscious decisions you've taken about how to behave and how to react to what life brings, and by the habits you've formed.

Bearing this out is the fact that the techniques in this book have been shown to increase levels of happiness in all sorts of people. How you think and what you do really does make a big difference.

Incidentally, there are all kinds of circumstances that people imagine will bring happiness, but which in fact do nothing of the sort. Material possessions, for example, won't do it – or at least not for long. All that happens is that we become used to our lovely new house, or car, or flat-screen TV. Fame won't bring happiness. Your level of intelligence matters not a jot.

Even money is no guarantee of well-being. Many of us fantasise about scooping a lottery jackpot, but whether lottery winners are any happier in the long run remains an open question (some studies suggest they may be; others have found no such evidence). Generally speaking, richer people are happier than poor people, but the difference between the two groups is small.

In fact, research suggests that, if you really want money to make you happy, you should spend it on other people. Perhaps the seventeenth-century scientist and philosopher Francis Bacon was right: 'Money is like muck: not good unless it be spread'.

This is all good news. Becoming happier doesn't depend on you moving to a bigger house, or winning the lottery, or becoming seventeen again. The changes you need to make are already firmly within your grasp.

WHY BE HAPPY?

In one sense, why we should want to be happy is obvious: because it feels so good. What more is there to say?

Well, as it happens, there's increasing evidence that happiness brings with it all kinds of previously unsuspected benefits. For instance, happy people are likely to enjoy better health. They live longer too. In fact, it's been suggested that happiness can make as much difference to your longevity as being a non-smoker, giving you an extra seven or so years of life.

As if that weren't enough, scientific research indicates that happy people tend to have more friends and stronger romantic relationships. And some psychologists believe happiness increases your creativity, imagination, analytical skills and productivity at work.

And yet we're willing to bet that you aren't looking to increase your happiness so that you can live longer or gain a promotion. What truly matters is not some future payoff, but your feelings in the here and now. Getting those feelings right is reward enough.

> " *What truly matters is not some future payoff, but your feelings in the here and now.* "

HOW TO USE THIS BOOK

As you'll have noticed, this is a relatively short book. It's also a practical book – an activity book, if you like.

These two characteristics are not unconnected. There's a vast body of work by psychologists on increasing happiness and combating unhappiness. But though that work informs what you'll read here, we've chosen to get right to the heart of the matter.

What this book offers are the proven scientific techniques you can use to increase your level of happiness. No waffle; just the key information you need to really make a difference to your mood. These techniques are based on the most up-to-date science, the results of research trials and clinical experience helping others.

What also makes this book different is our firm belief that the most successful route to happiness involves both calming our negative emotions and encouraging the positive. It's a two-pronged strategy.

Each chapter contains several practical exercises, suggestions and tips. That adds up to a lot of techniques! Don't feel that you have to adopt them all and all at once; in the beginning, aim to have a go at one technique per chapter.

Each technique is specifically designed to improve your mood. They've helped countless people around the world to become happier. Perhaps you're doubtful whether they'll work for you too. Maybe you won't fancy doing some of the activities. Some days you may feel too down or tired or stressed. But don't let these thoughts put you off.

For instance, in Chapter 3 we'll show you how important physical exercise is for happiness. You might feel you don't have the energy to go for a walk or a swim. Test this out by staying at home one time and then going out another. Chances are you'll discover that you feel happier, and have much more energy, after you've done some exercise. We want you to learn *from your own experience* that the techniques in this book are worth the effort.

And don't be bashful about asking friends and loved ones what they think happiness is and what makes them happy. Here are some of the suggestions we received when we asked around: 'Meeting a friend in a café'; 'Going for a walk in the countryside'; 'Watching a Laurel and Hardy film'; 'Reading my kids a bedtime story'; 'Dancing'; 'Playing squash'; 'Knitting'; 'Planning my next holiday'; 'Cooking a special meal for my partner'; 'Finding a spot in the sunshine'. What works for you?

We're almost ready to begin. Daunted? Apprehensive? Making any kind of significant change – even one as positive as increasing your happiness – can be unsettling. After all, you're leaving behind the familiar and heading off into the unknown. But this is a journey you're perfectly equipped to make.

We think you'll find it an interesting, enjoyable and satisfying one too. We all have habits we'd benefit from leaving behind. Here's your chance to replace them with more positive alternatives. As Einstein himself suggested, now's the time to begin seeing the world in a new light.

Remember that we're suggesting modest, gradual steps. One activity at a time. There's no need suddenly to turn your life on its head. Lasting change is built gradually and methodically, day by day. In due course, you'll be amazed at how far those small steps will have taken you. In fact, by simply making the decision to read this book you have begun to take action. You are taking control. That's already something to feel happy about!

MEASURING YOUR HAPPINESS

How happy would you say you are right now? That can be a surprisingly difficult question to answer with any precision. 'Fairly happy', 'Pretty happy' and 'So-so' are three typical, middling responses.

If you'd like to get a clearer sense of your own current happiness, you can take the following questionnaire. Don't worry if you don't feel like doing it right now: you can always come back to it at a later date, or not at all.

Happiness can be a slippery concept to measure. You might, for example, feel differently about various parts of your life, such as your work and your relationships. If that's the case, you could either give a general answer (a sort of average) or use the questionnaire to focus on one particular aspect of life. And if for whatever reason you find it tricky to answer specific questions, that's fine. Don't agonise about it; do the best you can and move on.

The Warwick–Edinburgh Mental Well-being Scale (WEMWBS)

The questionnaire contains some statements about feelings and thoughts. Base your answers on how you've been feeling over the past fortnight.

	NONE OF THE TIME	RARELY	SOME OF THE TIME	OFTEN	ALL OF THE TIME
I've been feeling optimistic about the future	1	2	3	4	5
I've been feeling useful	1	2	3	4	5
I've been feeling relaxed	1	2	3	4	5
I've been feeling interested in other people	1	2	3	4	5
I've had energy to spare	1	2	3	4	5
I've been dealing with problems well	1	2	3	4	5
I've been thinking clearly	1	2	3	4	5
I've been feeling good about myself	1	2	3	4	5
I've been feeling close to other people	1	2	3	4	5
I've been feeling confident	1	2	3	4	5
I've been able to make up my own mind about things	1	2	3	4	5

	NONE OF THE TIME	RARELY	SOME OF THE TIME	OFTEN	ALL OF THE TIME
I've been feeling loved	1	2	3	4	5
I've been interested in new things	1	2	3	4	5
I've been feeling cheerful	1	2	3	4	5
Scores					
Total score					

Source: © NHS Health Scotland, University of Warwick and University of Edinburgh, 2006. All rights reserved.

Now add up your scores: first for each of the columns, and then for the columns combined. The higher your score, the happier you probably are. If that seems a little vague, it's worth knowing that the average score is approximately 50 out of 70. You can find out more about the questionnaire at http://www. healthscotland.com/understanding/population/Measuring-positive-mental-health.aspx

Besides clarifying your feelings, there's another very important reason for completing this questionnaire. If you're setting out on a journey, you want to know that you're heading in the right direction. This questionnaire will help you do that. Make a note of your scores today. Then come back to the self-assessment in the coming weeks as you try out the happiness techniques in the following chapters and see just how much progress you've made. We're sure you'll be pleasantly surprised.

CHAPTER 2

Committing to happiness

Life is not easy for any of us. But what of that? We must have perseverance and above all confidence in ourselves.
MARIE CURIE

The very fact that you're reading this book shows that you are genuinely interested in becoming happier, and are curious about how you can do so. You've taken the crucial first step. Already you are moving forward. You're taking stock of where you are right now, and quite possibly viewing some parts of your daily life from a new perspective.

This chapter is all about taking that interest and curiosity to the next level. The objective is to develop and strengthen your motivation to become happier. But you don't have to rely simply on will power: we suggest a number of techniques and activities proven to help you achieve the right mindset for positive change.

ARE YOU READY TO COMMIT TO HAPPINESS?

Making a major change to the way you live your life – and deciding to increase your happiness is certainly one of those changes – usually follows a well-defined life cycle:

1 *Precontemplation*: We haven't acknowledged that we need or want to change.

2 *Contemplation*: We've accepted there may be an issue that needs tackling but we aren't yet ready to make a change.

3   *Preparation/Determination*: We're getting ready to change.

4   *Action/Will power*: We're changing our behaviour.

5   *Maintenance*: We're sticking with our new behaviour.
    In some cases, this stage is followed by:

6   *Relapse:* We fall back into our old habits.

Take a few moments to think about which stage you're at right now. If you're reading this book then you are at least at stage 2. If you're at stages 2 or 3, the exercises that follow in this chapter will help speed your progress to stages 4 and 5. (Chapter 11 will show you how to avoid stage 6.)

WEIGHING UP THE PROS AND CONS

A neat way to boost your motivation is to weigh up the pros and cons both of making a change and of sticking with the status quo. (It's a simple technique, but one that psychologists often use with clients when they're helping them prepare for change.) All you need is a piece of paper and a few minutes' thinking time. Sketch out a chart like the one below and fill in each of the columns.

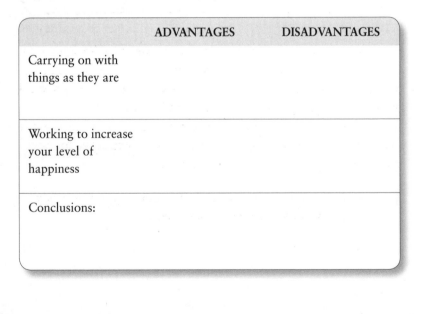

	ADVANTAGES	DISADVANTAGES
Carrying on with things as they are		
Working to increase your level of happiness		
Conclusions:		

This exercise is designed to help you discover how you really feel about change. What do you think is stopping you? What positives will drive you on to success? If you can pinpoint your motivation for becoming happier, you're much more likely to achieve it.

> **If you can pinpoint your motivation for becoming happier, you're much more likely to achieve it.**

Ask yourself: what are the advantages of aiming to increase your happiness? How will you feel when it happens? What will you do? What will change for the better?

Are there any disadvantages? Are you wondering if this might be too much effort? Are you sceptical about whether the techniques really will boost your happiness? Perhaps you're a bit worried about what you might be asked to do?

How about leaving things as they are? One of the advantages might be that the status quo, for all its drawbacks, is familiar and safe. And yet that might also be one of the disadvantages: the safe and familiar is no longer working for you. Change is required!

Sometimes it's difficult to obtain perspective on your own situation. So one useful tip for this exercise is to try to imagine what your friends and family would say. What advice would you give to someone in similar circumstances?

If this exercise has helped you crystallise your reasons for wanting to become happier, write them down in as snappy a form of words as you can. For example:

I want to move on from the status quo. Now I'm ready to change. I want to become the happier, better me.

Nothing is snappier than an acronym. So how about:

GHT: Give Happiness A Try, or
ICDI!: I Can Do It!

Put that piece of paper somewhere you can easily find it. You could also try jotting down your reasons for change on a card you can carry with you – that way, it'll always be there when you need it.

INSPIRATION

We all need role models – someone who can inspire us to become the person we dearly wish to be. Sometimes the lessons we learn are practical ('Ah, *that's* what I need to do in order to get promoted'). But often their influence is more general. They represent an ideal: a real, breathing demonstration of how we want to live our life. It won't be the same for everybody. And it may well be someone seemingly very 'ordinary' to anybody else.

Jenny is a thirty-four-year-old teacher. Here's what she told us about the inspirational figure in her life:

I've always thought of my grandmother as embodying the idea of a life well lived. She experienced her share of ups and downs, for sure. But she had a wonderful ability to come to terms with whatever life dealt her. I loved her calmness, her contentment, her gentleness. She didn't have a career. She never owned her own home. She never travelled outside this country; in fact, she hardly travelled anywhere at all. But none of these things mattered to her. Her priorities were her family, her friends, her garden. I don't think I've ever met someone who smiled as often – who was able to take so much satisfaction from the most ordinary events. She is the person I want most to be like. I often ask myself: how would Grandma behave in my situation? What would she say? What would she advise me to do? I feel so fortunate to have known her and to have been given such a fantastic role model.

Who inspires you? Whose story fills you with optimism, energy and joy? Whose image comes to mind when you hear the phrase 'a life well lived'? What is it about them that appeals so much? What changes would you need to make to your life to get closer to that ideal?

Perhaps like Jenny it's someone you've known personally. Maybe it's a figure from public life. Or perhaps you've been struck by a story you've come across in the media. Whoever it is that inspires you, spend a little time each day thinking about them. If it's someone currently in your life, keep those ties strong. If not, perhaps you can read about them, look at photographs, or savour memories.

You'll find this a great way of building your motivation for change. Not only that, it will keep you going during difficult times. Think of your inspiration as a beacon, always pointing the way to where you want to go. Keep that beacon in sight, and in time you're sure to get there.

> *Think of your inspiration as a beacon, always pointing the way to where you want to go.*

WRITE YOUR OWN TRIBUTE

In Chapter 1 we stated that happiness has four components:

- Pleasure
- Meaning
- Engagement
- Fewer negative emotions

Of course, this is a rather abstract view of happiness. It's like looking at an aerial photograph of the street where you live. (If you haven't already tried doing this on the Internet, give it a go: it's fun!) That aerial photograph gives you a fantastic high-level view of your local area, but what it doesn't reveal is the distinctive look and feel of your home. Similarly, while our definition of happiness captures the broad essence of the emotion, it doesn't describe the precise form happiness might take for you personally.

Perhaps you have a very clear idea of what contentment means for you. But if not, try writing your own tribute. Imagine that you are coming to the end of your life. What would you like to have achieved? How would you wish to be remembered? Keep in mind that you're not describing how you see yourself now, but rather what the ideal you might look like.

Here's an example written by Chris, a forty-year-old painter and decorator:

> He was a loyal friend, a devoted husband, a loving father and grandfather. He was kind, funny, patient, always looking on the bright side. The kind of person other people liked to be around.
>
> He enjoyed his work – the feeling he got when he saw how his efforts had transformed someone's home. He was proud of his practical ability. He played football for as long as he could, and then took up hiking and cycling. And he loved learning – he was always enrolled on one evening class or another. Later in life, he began teaching these classes and discovered that he enjoyed it enormously.
>
> On retirement, he became active in his local church. One of his most treasured memories was arriving there one Sunday with all six grandchildren. He saw himself as wonderfully fortunate: his life had been long, contented and useful. He would often remark: 'I have so much to be grateful for'.

This activity is a really effective method to help pinpoint what really matters to you – and what may be missing from your life. Once you realise what's lacking, you can begin to rectify that omission.

A POSITIVE MINDSET

The Olympic gold medallist Dame Kelly Holmes once commented: 'I knew I was stronger than I've ever been, but it's what goes on in your head that counts.'

Sports stars – and the specialist sports psychologists who advise them – know that what sets champions apart is not so much their natural ability, but the mindset they adopt in order to maximise that ability. It's good advice for us all: a positive mindset is the springboard for positive behaviour. You'll find it a huge help as you set about increasing your happiness. Remember: *it's what goes on in your head that counts.*

Here are some ways in which you can cultivate that positive mindset:

Set regular time aside to work with this book.
Making progress with anything is much easier if you work at it on a regular basis. If you're finding it tricky to balance the activities against your other responsibilities, try scheduling time for them in your diary. Simple as it sounds, this can be enough to help turn an aspiration into a firm commitment.

Stick to your guns!
Keep going, even if progress sometimes seems slow: you'll get there in the end. If you feel your resolve slipping, remind yourself why you're doing this in the first place – how much happier you'll feel and how much more enjoyable your life will be.

When the world says, 'Give up,'
Hope whispers, 'Try it one more time'.
ANON

Be willing to try things out.
You've already shown that you want to turn things around. To really push on, try to approach the various suggestions we make with an open and curious mind. You might not fancy trying some of the exercises; others might seem too 'obvious' to work. But if you give them a chance, they will help you to feel happier.

Back yourself to succeed.
Build your self-confidence by encouragement and rewards. Stay positive, remember how far you've come, and back yourself to push on to happiness. When you've completed an exercise or achieved a goal, celebrate your achievement. Congratulate yourself. Treat yourself to something you fancy – buy that treat or watch that film. Feel good about yourself: you deserve it.

Monitor your efforts.
Keep a notebook handy and jot down what you do from this book, what you learn and how you feel. It'll help you gain the distance to think clearly about your experiences. It will also show you just how much progress towards happiness you've made.

Enlist your support network.
How to be happy isn't a typical topic of conversation. Even as brothers, we'd never talked about it. But working on this book has prompted many discussions, both between the two of us and with friends and family, and every one of those conversations has proved helpful and thought-provoking.

So consider discussing happiness with those closest to you. You could start by keeping it abstract and general rather than personal – maybe you could mention something you've read or a story in the news that's got you thinking. But if the conversation goes well, you have the perfect opportunity to explain that you're taking practical steps to become happier. By doing so, you'll allow the people that matter to you to help you get where you want to go.

If you can build a support network, you provide yourself with a reliable source of practical help, encouragement and inspiration. They'll lift you when you're feeling down and celebrate with you when things are going well. And, as we mentioned in Chapter 1, you can ask your friends and family for their happiness tips. You'll probably find they suggest something you'd not thought of.

Then there's the fact that no one wants people they care about to see them as a quitter. Simply telling someone that you're working to increase your happiness makes it more likely that you'll stay the course.

> *telling someone that you're working to increase your happiness makes it more likely that you'll stay the course.*

But remember, if you're uncomfortable talking about these issues with friends and family, there's absolutely no need to do so. Perhaps you'll prefer to take it step by step, putting your toe in the metaphorical water to gauge how other people will react. Give it a try if you can: all the evidence suggests that it helps. But don't worry if it's not right for you. Becoming happier is within your control, whether anyone else knows what you're aiming for or not.

STEP BACK AND WEIGH UP

The activities we outline here are designed to help you become happier in all areas of your life – for example, your work, your leisure time, your relationships, your social life. Sometimes, though, you may need to stand back and really weigh up whether the situation calls for more drastic measures.

Imagine, for example, that you dislike your job. To be truly content in your working life, you may need either to quit or to modify your expectations. Emily chose the latter option. Ten years after leaving university, her dream of making a living designing and crafting jewellery felt further away than ever. She was becoming increasingly frustrated and depressed by the waitressing and administrative jobs she took to pay the rent.

After a lot of discussion with her friends, Emily came to a decision. Her solution was to accept these roles for what they were to her: a means to an end. My real work, she told herself, is my jewellery. This mental shift proved doubly effective. Not only did Emily find her day job much more bearable, she felt a renewed motivation to pursue her jewellery. (You'll find more on how to increase your happiness at work in Chapter 9.)

We hope this chapter will have helped you over a crucial hurdle. That hurdle separates desire and commitment: the desire to become happier and the commitment to make that happiness a reality.

The remaining chapters will set out exactly what you need to do to increase your happiness. We begin by looking at two important – but often overlooked – foundations for well-being: a good night's sleep and a healthy diet. This may sound obvious, but if you're tempted to skip the next chapter, please bear with us. You might be surprised to hear what science has to say...

CHAPTER 3

Getting the basics in place: improving your diet and sleep

The French writer Georges Perec once kept a record of everything he ate and drank for an entire year. He called it: 'Attempt at an Inventory of the Liquid and Solid Foodstuffs Ingurgitated by Me in the Course of the Year Nineteen Hundred and Seventy-four'. (If, like us, you struggle to remember what you ate for breakfast this morning, this remarkable feat is especially impressive…)

Let's imagine that you have done the same, but for just seven days. When you look back over your notes, you discover that during the week you have eaten:

- Lots of fruit and vegetables
- Plenty of wholewheat bread, pasta and rice
- Lots of fish
- Low-fat cheeses and yoghurt
- Dried fruit and unsalted nuts for your snacks
- Low-sugar, wholegrain breakfast cereals

You have drunk:

- Lots of water and fruit juice
- Fruit teas
- One cup of milky coffee each morning

You have avoided:

- Crisps
- Biscuits
- Ready meals
- Sweets
- Chocolate
- Red meat
- Cured meats and sausages
- Full-fat cheese
- Fried food
- Alcohol
- Fizzy drinks

Each night you have been in bed by ten. You have read for a few minutes before switching off the light. By ten forty-five you have been asleep, and you've slept right through till seven.

How do you think you'd feel after a week like this? Desperate for a glass of wine or a piece of chocolate, perhaps! But, that aside, probably feeling pretty good: rested, energetic, optimistic.

Now we're not suggesting you adopt such a spartan lifestyle. Food and drink are two of life's great pleasures. Enjoying an occasional late night in the company of friends certainly justifies some tiredness the next day.

But we do want to make the point that taking care of the basics, such as diet and sleep, can have a big positive impact on your emotions. Just as the mind can influence the body, so too can the condition of the body influence the mind. Look after your body and your efforts will be well rewarded, physically and psychologically.

> *" Look after your body and your*
> *efforts will be well rewarded,*
> *physically and psychologically. "*

This may seem like common sense. Perhaps your parents made the same point once or twice when you were a child! Maybe you're thinking: 'I know that.' However, though most of us are *aware* that we should be eating more healthily, getting more sleep and exercising regularly, these are the sort of lifestyle changes that it's easy to neglect. (Many of us have made short-lived New Year's resolutions on these topics!)

But if we're serious about increasing our well-being, we need to get these basics in place. The scientific evidence is clear: a healthy diet and plenty of good-quality sleep really can make you feel happier. One fascinating study followed more than 10,000 people in the UK between 2002 and 2004. The researchers found that those who made major improvements in their diet (even without increasing the amount of exercise they took) reported feeling much happier, calmer and more peaceful, and far less nervous and unhappy.

So in this chapter we talk you through what's best to eat and drink, and how to overcome any sleep problems you may be experiencing. Of course, making any kind of change can seem daunting when we're feeling down or stressed. But there's no need to turn your lifestyle upside down: even fairly modest changes will bring benefits. Whatever you can do, no matter how apparently insignificant, is a step in the right direction.

FIRST THINGS FIRST

Because your physical condition can exert such a big influence on your emotions, we recommend you start by booking check-ups with your doctor and dentist. Specifically, ask your doctor to check your blood pressure, body mass index and cholesterol levels. And if there's anything in particular that's concerning you, mention that too.

Chances are you'll have the satisfaction of walking away with a clean bill of health. But if there *are* any little niggles that need sorting out, now's the time. Being ill is not going to make you happier; feeling healthy, on the other hand, will certainly help. And you'll be rightly proud of yourself to have taken action.

If you're a smoker, think seriously about stopping. You won't need us to point out the health problems associated with smoking. In the short term, smoking may be a pleasure; in the long term, it's likely to bring illness and unhappiness. The sense of achievement you'll feel when you quit will be a fantastic reward in itself. If you'd like guidance on giving up smoking, have a chat with your GP.

IMPROVING YOUR DIET

> *We are indeed much more than what we eat, but what we eat can nevertheless help us to be much more than what we are.*
> ADELLE DAVIS, PIONEERING US NUTRITIONIST

What exactly *is* a healthy diet? The fact that there are hundreds of books on the topic might suggest that nutrition is a complex business. In fact, positive nutrition is simple – so simple that it can be summed up in just ten guidelines.

If you want to make changes to your diet, do it gradually. Discarding habits you've built up over several years is best tackled step by step. So aim to introduce one change per week – for example, eating more oily fish or opting for a healthier breakfast cereal.

> **If you want to make changes to your diet, do it gradually.**

1   **Base your meals around starchy foods.** Starchy foods like bread, cereals, rice, pasta, and potatoes should make up about a third of our daily diet. They're a great source of energy, and are rich in fibre, calcium, iron and B vitamins. Go for wholewheat or wholegrain varieties: they contain more fibre and other nutrients.

2   **Eat lots of fruit and vegetables.** Try to eat at least five portions of fruit and vegetables a day. If you're not sure how much a portion is, visit www.nhs.uk and search for '5 a day'.

3   **Eat more fish.** Fish contains lots of protein, minerals and vitamins. Oily fish are rich in the omega 3 fatty acids that can help keep our hearts healthy. Aim to eat fish at least twice a week – and make sure that one of those is an oily fish like salmon, mackerel, trout, herring, fresh tuna (not tinned), sardines, pilchards and eels. Women who might want to become pregnant at some stage shouldn't eat more than two portions of oily fish a week; the limit otherwise is four.

4   **Cut down on saturated fat.** We all need some fat in our diet, but be wary of saturated fat, which can increase the amount of cholesterol in our blood and escalate the risk of heart disease. Unsaturated fat, on the other hand, *lowers* cholesterol.

Foods high in *saturated fat* include meat pies, sausages, cured meats, hard cheese, butter and lard, pastry, cakes and biscuits, cream, soured cream and crème fraîche. Good sources of *unsaturated fat* are vegetable oils (including sunflower, rapeseed and olive oil), oily fish, avocados, nuts and seeds.

5   **Eat less sugar.** Sugary foods and drinks cause tooth decay and are high in calories. Check the labels and watch out for foods that contain more than 5g of sugar per 100g.

6   **Reduce your salt intake to no more than 6 grams a day.** Eating too much salt increases our chances of having a

stroke or developing heart disease. Seventy-five per cent of the salt we eat is already in the food we buy. So again, check the label and go for low-salt options – less than 0.3g of salt per 100g.

7   **Drink plenty of water.** Aim to drink 1.2 litres of fluid every day to prevent dehydration. Water's best, but other drinks count too – such as tea or fruit juice. Avoid sugary drinks though.

8   **Don't overdo the caffeine.** There are now more than 10,000 chain coffee shops in the UK, not to mention countless independent cafés: proof, if proof were needed, of the nation's passion for coffee. For increasing numbers of people, coffee is an essential part of the daily routine – and a reliable source of great pleasure.

If you love your coffee there's no need to deprive yourself of that pleasure. But be aware that drinking a lot of coffee can raise your blood pressure, trigger feelings of anxiety or irritation, and interfere with your sleep – all of which will have a negative effect on your happiness. Remember too that caffeine is also found in tea, and many cola and energy drinks.

9   **Watch your alcohol intake.** Alcohol isn't usually a problem provided we don't drink too much. Women shouldn't regularly drink more than 2–3 units per day; for men the limit is 3–4 units a day. More than this on a regular basis can lead to health problems. Alcohol is also high in calories – cutting back is a great way to lose weight.

10 **Don't skip breakfast.** Missing breakfast might seem like a sensible slimming technique, but it usually has the opposite effect. Because we're ravenous midway through the morning, we fill the gap with tasty snacks like biscuits, pastries and chocolate, thereby consuming far more calories than we would have done if we had enjoyed a healthy breakfast. Eat *regular* meals, including a nutritious breakfast – wholegrain cereal and fruit, for instance – and stave off the snack attack!

IMPROVING YOUR SLEEP

Most of us know from experience that sleep – and sleeplessness – can have a dramatic effect on our mood. And many research studies confirm this: sleeping poorly can make us anxious, depressed and irritable. In contrast, there's a clear link between good sleep and happiness, particularly pleasure and engagement. Clinical studies show that tackling sleep problems leads to an improvement in mood. And yet, the stresses and strains of modern life mean that increasing numbers of people aren't getting the sleep they require.

Make sleep a priority. People vary in how much they need, but most adults function best on at least seven or eight hours. Just as important as quantity, however, is the quality of your sleep. Eight hours in bed at night doesn't necessarily mean eight hours of deep and invigorating rest.

> " *as important as quantity, however,*
> *is the quality of your sleep.* "

It's normal to have times when you don't sleep as well as you'd like, but how can you tell whether you have a real sleep problem? The following questionnaire is a good place to start. It assesses whether you may be suffering from insomnia, the most common type of sleep problem. Insomnia is a general term for a number of issues:

- Struggling to fall asleep
- Finding it hard to stay asleep
- Not having enough sleep
- Not experiencing enough good-quality sleep

PART A	NOT AT ALL	SOMEWHAT	QUITE A LOT	VERY MUCH
1. I find it difficult to fall asleep.	1	2	3	4
2. Thoughts go through my head and keep me awake.	1	2	3	4
3. I worry and find it hard to relax.	1	2	3	4
4. I wake up during the night.	1	2	3	4
5. After waking up during the night, I fall asleep slowly.	1	2	3	4
6. I wake up early and cannot get back to sleep.	1	2	3	4
7. I sleep lightly.	1	2	3	4
8. I sleep too little.	1	2	3	4
9. Generally, I sleep badly.	1	2	3	4
Total score for Part A:				

PART B	NOT AT ALL	SOMEWHAT	QUITE A LOT	VERY MUCH
1. I feel tired when I get up.	1	2	3	4
2. I feel sleepy during the day and struggle to remain alert.	1	2	3	4
3. I would like to have more energy during the day.	1	2	3	4
4. People tell me I'm easily irritated.	1	2	3	4
5. I have difficulty concentrating at work or school.	1	2	3	4
6. I worry whether I sleep enough.	1	2	3	4
7. I have sleep attacks (i.e. suddenly feeling very sleepy) during the day.	1	2	3	4
Total score for Part B:				

Source: Spoormaker, V.I., van den Bout, J., Klip, E.C., 'Initial validation of the SLEEP-50 questionnaire', *Behavioural Sleep Medicine*, 3, 227–46 (2005)
© Taylor & Francis Group (http://www.informaworld.com)

Now add up your scores for Parts A and B. You may be suffering from insomnia if you've scored:

- 14–18 on Part A **and**
- 11–14 on Part B

Severe (or *clinical*) insomnia is likely if you've scored:

- 19 or more on Part A **and**
- 19 or more on Part B

IMPROVING YOUR SLEEP

> *Blessed be whoever invented sleep, the mantle that covers all human thought, the food that satisfies hunger, the water that quenches thirst, the fire that warms the cold, the cold that cools down ardour, and, finally, the general coin with which all things are bought, the scale and the balance that make the shepherd equal to the king, and the simple man equal to the wise.* CERVANTES, DON QUIXOTE

To improve your sleep, try these five techniques:

Exercise every day.
It's simple: exercise tires us out, and if we're tired, we're likely to sleep better.

Avoid caffeine, alcohol and nicotine in the evening.

Develop a relaxing evening routine.
At least half an hour before bedtime, begin winding down. Do something calm and restful: perhaps a warm bath or some time reading or listening to gentle music.

Have a bedtime snack.
A little food about thirty minutes before bed can help with sleep. Go for something healthy and relatively plain: a glass of milk, a banana, or perhaps a piece of wholewheat toast.

Get your bedroom right for sleep.
That means a comfortable bed, and a room that's quiet, dark and your preferred temperature (around 18°C is usually ideal).

These steps should do the trick, but if your insomnia hasn't improved it's time to move on to stage 2. Within a few days of adopting the following guidelines, you should notice a big improvement in your sleep.

Resist the temptation to lie in, and cut out daytime naps
– you'll only find it harder to fall asleep at night.

Only go to bed when you're tired.
Switch off the light as soon as you're comfortable.

Learn to associate your bed with sleep.
Don't use it, say, for reading, eating, watching TV, or writing a diary. (Sex is permissible, though, because it generally leaves us feeling sleepy.)

Don't let bedtime be worry time.
Instead, try setting aside twenty minutes earlier in the evening to think through your problems. If you find yourself worrying while you're in bed, jot the thought down on a piece of paper ready for tomorrow's worry session and let it go for the night.

If you haven't fallen asleep within twenty minutes, get up and do something relaxing.
It's the same if you wake up in the night: if you haven't fallen back to sleep after twenty minutes, get up and only go back to bed when you're feeling tired.

WHAT IF YOU'RE SLEEPING TOO MUCH?

Insomnia is sleeplessness. Some people, though, seem to have the opposite problem: too much sleep. Whatever time the alarm goes is too early: they simply ignore it and go back to sleep.

Sometimes oversleeping is a by-product of insomnia – a way of catching up on a bad night's sleep. For other people, it can be a sign that they're feeling particularly down (see Chapter 10 for more on this).

Whatever the cause, it's best to follow the guidelines above for achieving regular, good-quality sleep. Make sure you have something to get up in the morning for – whether that be arriving at work on time, getting the kids off to school, going for a swim, or meeting a friend. Don't interpret your sleepiness as a sign that you need more rest.

These steps will help you relearn the necessary habit of getting up in the morning. Of course, we can't guarantee that you'll greet the morning alarm with glee, but by the time it sounds you will at least have enjoyed a good night's sleep!

Making even modest improvements to your diet and sleep habits will soon pay dividends. So go for it. You'll be amazed at how much more positive you feel.

CHAPTER 4
Activities for happiness

'Joy's soul', wrote Shakespeare in *Troilus and Cressida*, 'lies in the doing.' For those of us who want to become happier, this is an absolutely crucial – and wonderfully empowering – message. This is especially so because Shakespeare's insight is backed up by contemporary science: what we *do* can have a profound effect on the way we *feel*.

But if we're choosing activities to increase our happiness, which ones should we go for?

FIVE A DAY FOR HAPPINESS

A few years back the UK government commissioned a report into the mental health of the nation, and what could be done to improve it. After consultations with more than 400 experts, the report advocated a '5 a day' programme for well-being. Here are the five recommended types of activity:

- Connect
- Be active
- Be curious
- Learn
- Give

We'll look at each of these in more detail shortly. But first let's spend a moment thinking about that word 'activity'.

Do we mean that you can't be happy dozing on the sofa or watching your favourite soap opera? No, we certainly don't! Everyone needs down time, but to really keep ourselves psychologically healthy, all the evidence suggests that this kind of passive relaxation needs to be balanced by a wide range of other activities – which is where the '5 a day' come in.

Connect

> Let us be grateful to people who make us happy: they
> are the charming gardeners who make our souls blossom.
> MARCEL PROUST

Connecting is all about building relationships with other people – family, friends, colleagues and neighbours. When scientists analyse the characteristics of happy people, it's always the quality of their relationships that stands out. Happy folk have more friends, and stronger intimate relationships, than unhappy individuals.

> " *Happy folk have more friends*
> *than unhappy individuals.* "

But this does *not* mean that happiness depends on having a devoted spouse, picture-book extended family and dozens of friends. Quality is more important than quantity. With just a few close friends you can turn to, you'll be absolutely fine.

In fact, it's not even necessary for all of those friends to be human! Owning a pet, research suggests, both boosts positive feelings and helps us cope with negative emotions such as stress and anxiety.

Remember the four components of happiness we identified in Chapter 1:

● Pleasure

● Meaning

● Engagement

● Fewer negative emotions

Our relationships can supply all of those components. For example, think back to the last time you laughed out loud: we're willing to bet you weren't alone. Spending time with other people offers lots of opportunities for fun – or, to use the jargon, hedonic pleasure.

Relationships can also be a rich source of meaning in our lives – taking us out of ourselves and into a wider community, whether that be family, your team at work, or perhaps a club or voluntary organisation.

When it comes to activities that generate engagement (or 'flow'), doing them with others is proven to be even better than doing them alone. For example, one experiment had people playing a ball game either alone or with another person. The levels of flow were the same, but playing the game with another person was found to be more enjoyable.

Moreover, there's lots of research to suggest that strong relationships don't just boost positive emotions; they also help us cope with negative feelings.

In fact, relationships are so important for happiness that we've devoted a whole chapter to them (see Chapter 8).

Be active

Physical exercise isn't simply good for your body, it's also a great way to build positive emotions. In the previous chapter we highlighted the impact a healthy diet and plenty of good-quality sleep can have on your happiness. It's just the same with exercise: look after your body and you'll also be caring for your mind.

Aim for at least 30 minutes of exercise several times a week. If you're starting from zero and that's too daunting, try every other day and build up from there. Ideally, your exercise should make your heartbeat and breathing a little faster than normal. You'll feel warm and may well work up a sweat. Aerobic activities like brisk walking, swimming, jogging, dancing and tennis are especially beneficial but, whatever you go for, make sure it's something you really enjoy.

If sport isn't your thing, remember that any activity that gets your cardiovascular system working is perfect – that might be gardening, playing with the children, vacuuming the house, or walking briskly to the shops. What you do is much less important than the physical effects produced by that activity.

One tried and tested way of spicing up an exercise plan is to do it with other people. And it's not just more enjoyable; you're more likely to turn up for your exercise session if you know someone else is expecting you. So could you persuade a friend to join you for a walk or swim or game of badminton? Is there an exercise class you could attend?

Aim to build exercise into your daily routine – that way you'll get your exercise without really noticing it. For example, rather than driving to work, walk or cycle instead. Try getting off the bus a couple of stops early and walking the rest of the way. If you can vary your route, so much the better: you're less likely to become bored.

Simply getting outside can provide a real boost to your system, especially if the weather is good. And spending time in the countryside provides a reliable pick-me-up. Given this, why not try hiking? Fresh air, beautiful scenery, brilliant exercise: hiking has it all!

> **Simply getting outside can provide a real boost to your system**

Exercise is a great way to experience engagement or flow – the feeling of being so completely focused on the task at hand that you lose all self-awareness. And engagement, as we saw in Chapter 1, is a core component of happiness.

But hang on a minute, you might be thinking: I can easily lose myself in a TV programme or a trashy novel. Doesn't that tick the engagement box?

The answer is that real flow – the sort we get from playing sports, or working on a puzzle, or learning a musical instrument – happens when we're being *challenged*. We have to be working near the limit of our skills and knowledge. If the activity is too easy, we risk boredom; if it's too difficult, we become frustrated. TV and trashy novels can give us pleasure – and that's not to be sniffed at – but they can't provide the kind of deep satisfaction that real flow activities bring.

Be curious

'I think, at a child's birth, if a mother could ask a fairy godmother to endow it with the most useful gift, that gift should be curiosity', wrote author, activist and First Lady of the US Eleanor Roosevelt.

Curiosity and love of life go hand in hand. Think of the happy people you know. We bet they're brimming with inquisitiveness, always interested in what life has to offer. Doubtless they're able to find something to delight and intrigue in even the most ordinary situations, savouring details that often pass the rest of us by: the colour of a tree's leaves, perhaps, the taste of a biscuit, or the pleasure of a few moments' conversation with a stranger.

> *Curiosity and love of life*
> *go hand in hand.*

Cultivate your curiosity. Take the time to notice what's going on around you; the appearance of the objects and people nearby; the sensations in your body. Allow yourself to wonder why something is the way it is. Ask yourself the questions we all normally take for granted. Where might that person be going? Why is the bird perching on the telephone wire? What is the most appealing thing you can see when you look around you – and what makes it so attractive? By doing so, you'll be truly *engaging* with your world. You'll discover that there's much more to enjoy than you ever suspected.

Learn

> *The excitement of learning separates youth from old age.*
> *As long as you are learning you're not old.* ROSALYN SUSSMAN
> YALOW (1921–2011), NOBEL PRIZE-WINNING MEDICAL PHYSICIST

Whether it's a new language or learning to sail, first aid or playing the guitar, learning a new skill is a proven route to satisfaction, fun and self-confidence.

It doesn't matter what you're learning; happiness arises from your awareness that you're becoming increasingly proficient at an activity, whatever that might be. You're moving forward: sticking to your task and developing new skills.

If you're studying alongside other people, you have the fun of social contact. And as if that weren't enough, learning is also a really effective way of generating engagement: the challenge of mastering the skill or subject area is so compelling that your self-awareness will vanish.

Give

> *If you desire an hour's happiness, take a nap. If you desire*
> *a day's happiness, go fishing. If you desire a month's*
> *happiness, get married. If you desire a year's happiness,*
> *inherit a fortune. If you desire a lifetime's happiness, help*
> *someone else.* CHINESE PROVERB

Imagine that tomorrow you treat yourself to a small box of exquisite homemade chocolates, and that you eat those chocs while watching your favourite television programme. The following day you notice a harassed mother leaving the supermarket. She is trying to push her overladen trolley to the car park. Meanwhile, her two toddlers are wailing in protest at being removed from the Bob the Builder ride positioned so helpfully in the supermarket entrance. You offer to take care of the trolley and help unload its contents into her car.

Which of these two acts is likely to bring you the most happiness: eating the chocolates and watching TV or helping the stressed mum?

When psychologists have run a similar experiment, the participants generally find that helping others gives them more satisfaction than, say, a box of chocolates. In other words, philanthropy beats fun. Meaning aces hedonistic pleasure.

This isn't to say that pleasure is unimportant; as we've seen, it's a vital component of happiness. But study after study has found that helping others – giving our time, attention and energy – is a crucial element of well-being. For example, researchers in Germany who followed the fortunes of thousands of people over several years found that those who were committed to helping other people were significantly happier – as were those who prioritised family, friends and social and political activities. (On the other hand, people driven by material rewards and job success were relatively unhappy.)

Try it yourself: one day hedonistic pleasure, the next day helping another person. Which feels best and how long does the happiness last?

Now you're aware of the key types of activity, you can start thinking about specific examples to build into your own routine. The following exercises will help you to do this, but don't forget to talk to friends and family too. You're bound to generate lots of ideas that way. And try surfing the web for possible activities.

You might be nervous about signing up for a class, or trying something you've never done before. But remember that these feelings are absolutely normal and will soon pass. You've risen to challenges like this in the past and you can do so again. It's easier if you remind yourself why you're doing it; if you keep in mind that any temporary feelings of anxiety will quickly be replaced by a sense of pride, pleasure and achievement.

Ask a friend along for support – it's usually more enjoyable to do things with other people than alone. Reward yourself for your courage and determination. And remember that joining a club or class isn't the only way to take up a new activity – there are books, CDs and Internet materials to help you master pretty much any activity you can think of.

BUILDING ON YOUR STRENGTHS AND VALUES

Each of us possesses *strengths* (what we're good at) and *values* (what we believe is important). When you're thinking about the kind of activities you might like to get involved in or simply have a go at, it's a good idea to take your strengths and values into account.

Psychologists have done a lot of work on how strengths and values contribute to happiness. Below, for example, is a list of character strengths identified by the Values in Action (VIA) Institute. Each of them is thought to aid well-being.

Creativity	Curiosity
Love of learning	Judgement/critical thinking/ open-mindedness
Perspective/wisdom	Honesty/authenticity/integrity
Bravery	Perseverance
Zest/energy	Kindness

Love	Social intelligence (being sensitive to other people's needs and desires)
Fairness	Leadership
Teamwork	Forgiveness/mercy
Modesty/humility	Prudence
Self-regulation (self-discipline)	Appreciation of beauty and excellence
Gratitude	Hope
Humour	Religiousness/spirituality

Source: From Peterson, P. and Seligman, M., *Character Strengths and Virtues: A Handbook Classification* (OUP USA, 2004), Copyright 2004 VIA Institute on Character (www.viacharacter.org)

The list isn't exhaustive, but it does give a flavour of what we mean when we talk about strengths.

If you'd like to assess your own strengths, take the VIA Survey at www.viasurvey.org

When it comes to values, here's what people surveyed in seventy countries rank as most important:

- Achievement
- Caring for others
- Respect for others
- Pleasure
- Power
- Security and safety
- Independence and freedom
- Excitement, variety, challenge
- Tradition
- Equality and justice

When we're thinking about activities to pursue, it's logical to choose those that are in harmony with your values. If excitement is what really matters to you, for instance, you'd probably be best advised to get your physical exercise mountain-biking or skateboarding rather than jogging!

Similarly, many experts suggest that, to become happier, we should aim to fill our lives with activities that build on our natural – or 'signature' – strengths. If you're creative, for example, look for new ways to use that strength. If you're intrigued by spiritual matters, consider what you can do to develop that interest. And if you're never happier than when researching a new subject, make learning a core part of your life.

> *It is never too late to be who you might have been.*
> GEORGE ELIOT

This makes perfect sense. Doing something well is wonderfully satisfying. Competence feels great. And because it feels great, we're much more likely to keep going with a new activity that plays to our strengths.

On the other hand, don't give up on an activity because it doesn't seem to fit well with your strengths. For example, you may feel that you're not particularly curious. Perhaps you find social situations difficult. Maybe you've always believed you don't have much get up and go. Don't let this stop you from developing your interest in the world, or building strong relationships, or getting out there and taking up a new form of exercise.

Believe in yourself. You can achieve so much more than you think, or than others may have led you to believe. Take a big, bold step outside your comfort zone – you'll be astonished at what you can achieve.

> ❝ *Believe in yourself. You can achieve*
> *so much more than you think* ❞

WHICH ACTIVITIES HAVE YOU ENJOYED IN THE PAST?

Here's an exercise to help identify the activities that make you happy. It involves reflecting on what's worked for you in the past. Start by jotting down the '5 a day' categories:

- Connect
- Be active
- Be curious
- Learn
- Give

Now, for each category, think back to an example in your own life – a time when you were truly happy. Here's what Lorna, a fifty-year-old office administrator, came up with:

Connect: Definitely the salsa dancing class I joined a few years back. I met so many lovely people – I'm still in touch with lots of the girls even after all this time. I was a bit shy about signing up, but I'm so glad I did.

Be active: The salsa dancing again: I felt so fit. What a fabulous workout!

Be curious: I kept a diary for a while. I wanted to capture what my children were like when they were little. Because I knew I'd have to write something at the end of each day, I paid a lot more attention to what was going on. I noticed lots of little details that I wouldn't have paid attention to otherwise. Life seemed so much fuller.

Learn: I really enjoyed my evening classes in print-making and line-drawing. It was fascinating learning about the techniques and then trying them out. It really fuelled my curiosity, so perhaps I should have put this under that heading too. And the classes were another great way to meet people, so that's 'Connect' again!

Give: Helping out at school when my children were young. I used to listen to the kids reading and accompany them on trips. I even filled in as a dinner lady when someone was on maternity leave. It was so satisfying to be involved and to feel you were contributing, even in a small way, to the education and welfare of the children.

After completing this exercise, pick one of the activities you've enjoyed in the past. Use it as inspiration for the New You. Lorna decided to enrol in a watercolour painting class. Which pleasure will you rediscover?

Remembering activities you've enjoyed in the past might not come easily. You may have to go back quite a long way. But that's fine: even recalling something you enjoyed many years ago could spark an idea for a current activity. If you used to enjoy cricket as a teenager, then even decades later you could look into local cricket clubs to see whether they have a practice night or informal 'play for fun' teams. Perhaps you enjoyed art or acting at school – why not explore ways of reviving those lost pleasures?

BRAINSTORMING ACTIVITIES FOR HAPPINESS

To help you think of an activity you'll enjoy, ask yourself these questions:

● What could I do for an afternoon that I'd really find fun or satisfying?

● What could I do for an hour?

● Is there something good I could plan to do one weekend?

● What can I do that costs money?

● What can I do for free?

● What could I do that will really stimulate my mind?

● What would give me a sense of achievement?

● Is there a course or evening class I'd find interesting?

- What physical activity would I like to do?
- What about learning a practical skill?
- If a friend was visiting, what would I suggest we do?
- Do I want to meet new people?
- Do I want to make new friends?
- What enjoyable activity could I do on my own?
- What could I do at home?
- Where would I like to go?
- What could I do that I've never done before?
- What have I enjoyed doing in the past?
- Are there any interesting events or activities listed in the paper?
- Could I just get some lists of what classes are available, to get ideas?
- Where else could I look for inspiration? The library? Tourist Information?
- How about voluntary work?

COMPILING YOUR ACTIVITIES DIARY

You're now familiar with the five types of activity that lead to happiness. You've identified examples that have brought you happiness in the past, considered how you can build on your strengths and values, and brainstormed with friends and family.

Now it's time to think about which activities to prioritise and how they'll fit with your week.

To help you decide, keep an activities diary for a week. It'll only take a few minutes each day; there's no need to write hundreds of words. Just make a brief note of what you were doing at a particular time, and how you were feeling. Here's a format you could use:

TIME	WHAT WAS I DOING?	HOW WAS I FEELING?
8.00–9.00am		
9.00–10.00am		
10.00–11.00am		
11.00–12.00pm		
12.00–1.00pm		
1.00–2.00pm		
2.00–3.00pm		
3.00–4.00pm		
4.00–5.00pm		
5.00–6.00pm		
6.00–7.00pm		
7.00–8.00pm		
8.00–9.00pm		
9.00–10.00pm		
10.00–11.00pm		

At the end of the week, look back through your diary. Ask yourself:

- Which activities did I enjoy?
- Which activities were less enjoyable for me?
- Which of the '5 a day' activities for happiness did I do a lot of? Which ones did I spend least time on?

Spend some time thinking about these questions and you'll soon notice the patterns. The links between your activities and your emotions will suddenly become clear. Then you can start planning your week to boost your happiness. Here's how:

- Aim to do more of the things that bring you happiness, though be wary of short-term kicks such as chocolate and alcohol. These fleeting pleasures are fine in moderation, but don't base your strategy for happiness on them.

- Either reduce the amount of time you spend doing the things you don't like or, if that's unrealistic, find ways to make them more enjoyable. For example, you might find the morning commute to work stressful and unpleasant. Can you improve it by, say, arranging to travel with a friend or using the time to learn a new skill?

- Prioritise the '5 a day' activities that you're currently light on. Add one target activity to your week: a few minutes a day or an hour or two a week is fine to begin with. For example, if you notice you're not as physically active as you'd like, try a brisk twenty-minute walk each day or a weekly swim.

- Once you've incorporated this new activity into your routine, you can gradually increase the amount of time you devote to it, or add another activity.

- Reward yourself for your efforts. Even if you're struggling to do as much as you'd like, remember that everything you achieve is a bonus, a step in the right direction.

It's a good idea to update your activities diary at the beginning of each month. You'll be able to track how you've reshaped your activities, and increased your happiness.

SETTING YOUR HAPPINESS GOALS

Armed with your insights from the exercises in this chapter, you can set yourself some *happiness goals*. It's often said that goals are dreams with deadlines. They help to make things happen instead of just thinking about them in a vague way.

Try to identify at least one goal for each of the '5 a day' activities. For example:

- *Connect*: Go to the cinema once a fortnight with my best friend.

- *Be active*: Take up badminton again.

- *Be curious*: Spend ten minutes each day thinking about my surroundings, what I'm doing, and how my body feels.

- *Learn*: Find out how my car works and how to carry out basic maintenance and repairs.

- *Give:* Spend one day a month volunteering for my favourite charity.

Once you've selected your high-level goals, break them down into smaller subgoals. For instance, a goal to play badminton might involve researching possible venues; choosing a playing partner; fixing a regular time, and so on.

Each time you achieve one of these subgoals, celebrate with a little treat. You deserve to have your efforts recognised and rewarded.

Working towards five goals at once is pretty ambitious, of course, so start with just one. When you feel comfortable with the progress you've made, consider beginning another from your list.

TIPS FOR SUCCESS

As you work towards fulfilling your happiness goals, remember these tips for success:

- **Schedule activities in advance.** It's easy for other commitments to crowd out the things we want to do for ourself. So plan your activities in advance, and add them to your diary. No one likes missing an appointment – even an appointment with yourself!

- **Make your new activities part of your routine.** When an activity has really taken root in our life we don't have to think about doing it. It seems as normal as our other habits.

  That's what you're aiming for when you start your new activities. It'll take time, for sure, but you can accelerate the process by making sure you do whatever it is often and regularly. Before long it'll seem natural that you go out for a run on Sundays, Tuesdays and Thursdays, or that you volunteer at your local hospice on the last Saturday of each month.

- **Keep it fresh.** Planning your goals, and making your new activities part of your routine, is a really effective way of getting things done. But watch out for staleness. If you're doing something just because it's there in your schedule rather than providing enjoyment, it's time to shake things up. If it's a chore, it's not going to make you happy. And happiness, of course, is what it's all about.

  If you find yourself in this situation, think about varying your routine, and perhaps changing the activity in question. For example, if you're a runner, maybe alter your route or begin running with other people. Perhaps consider swapping a run for a swim or cycle. Aim to keep it fun by keeping it fresh.

- **Join the club!** Adding a new activity to a busy schedule can be tough. But it's much easier – and much more fun – if you're doing that activity with friends or colleagues, rather than alone.

  If your goal is to learn how to cook, for example, think about joining a class, or having a friend or family member teach you, rather than trying to piece it all together yourself from recipe books. If you want to become more physically active, consider joining a swimming or cycling club. Chances are you'll not only achieve your goal, you'll make new friends doing so.

MINI-ACTIVITIES FOR DAILY HAPPINESS

This chapter has focused on helping you introduce new activities to your week. But you can boost your happiness simply by adding a few 'mini-activities' to your day.

Each morning – perhaps while you're in the shower or commuting to work – think of five positive things you can do that day. Select one for each of the 5 a day categories. For example:

● Connect: Chat to someone at coffee break.

● Be active: Go for a walk at lunchtime.

● Curiosity: Spend a few moments looking at something I've not noticed before at work.

● Learn: Discover the meaning of one new word.

● Give: Ask a colleague whether I can help them.

At the end of the day, review your progress. How many of these mini-activities can you tick off?

Remember: by ensuring your week includes the right type of activities, you can radically boost your level of happiness. There's no need to go overboard. It isn't necessary for you to suddenly turn your whole routine upside down. Small steps in the right direction will soon produce amazing results.

> " *by ensuring your week includes the right type of activities, you can radically boost your level of happiness.* "

Now let's turn our attention to another key influence on our happiness: our thoughts. We'll begin in the following chapter by explaining what you can do to overcome negative emotions.

CHAPTER 5

Calming negative thoughts

Life is full of ups and downs. But, strange though it may seem, research has shown that it isn't events that have the biggest influence on our emotions: it's the way we *react* to those events. As the seventeenth-century poet John Milton wrote:

> The mind is its own place, and in itself
> Can Make a Heaven of Hell, a Hell of Heaven

Think about it. Don't you know someone who is capable of finding the negative in even the most positive situation? On the other hand, we bet you can think of a person who can find something to smile about during even the toughest of times.

What this means is that we all have at our disposal an incredibly powerful tool to boost our happiness. That tool is our mind. To be content, we don't have to rely on 'good' things happening to us; we can discover the good anywhere we look. We can enjoy well-being pretty much wherever we happen to find ourselves, but we have to know how to use that tool. We must learn how to tame our negative thoughts, and increase the power of our positive thoughts. When we can do this, happiness will always be within our grasp.

This chapter focuses on the first part of the equation: the techniques we can use to calm our negative thoughts.

EXPRESS YOURSELF

One tried-and-tested technique to tackle negative thoughts and feelings is to write about them. Psychologists call this *expressive writing*, and it's been associated with a host of benefits, from greater happiness to an enhanced immune system.

Aim to write for twenty minutes three to four times each week. The trick is not to analyse your thoughts and feelings; simply *describe* them. Don't try to explain or judge them – and definitely don't worry about them. Instead, imagine you are writing a precise, factual report so that another person can understand exactly how you've been thinking and feeling.

Amazing as it seems, you'll discover that merely writing your thoughts down is enough to rob them of their power. When we're worried about something, we don't really get to grips with our feelings. Instead, our thoughts simply circulate repetitively through our mind. But writing those thoughts down helps our brain process our emotions.

> " *merely writing your thoughts down is enough to rob them of their power.* "

Here's what Susie, a twenty-three-year-old trainee physiotherapist, said about her experience of expressive writing:

It's a very strange, very wonderful thing. Writing really does help. It's as if my worries can't exist in two places at once. Once they're on paper, they can't be in my head. Sometimes I even throw the paper away: that feels great – I'm wishing my bad thoughts good riddance! And if I do have a bad thought at any point, I look forward to writing it out later. I feel more in control.

OVERCOMING WORRY

Everyone worries from time to time: it's a normal part of life. But if worrying is getting you down, it's time to take action. Here's how:

- **Identify what you think is positive about worrying – and challenge it.**

  Chances are, you're fully aware of the negative aspects of worrying – the anxiety, the monotony, the exhausting restlessness – but what you may be less conscious of are your positive beliefs about worry.

  Though we may be only dimly aware of it, worry is often fuelled by the sense that it somehow helps us. For example, people often believe deep down that worrying allows them to anticipate and solve problems; that it provides the motivation necessary to tackle those problems; or that it prepares them for the worst if a solution can't be found. They may even feel that worrying about an event might prevent it happening.

  These positive beliefs aren't helpful, so we need to loosen their grip. The best way to do this is simply to become aware of them and then to challenge them. Spend a few moments thinking through your motivation for worrying. What do you think are the benefits? How do you believe worrying helps you? Now think back to your recent experiences with worry: have those benefits materialised? Has worrying really helped? Would the situation have worked out differently if you hadn't spent all that time worrying?

- **Don't panic!** Worry *about* worry can be a problem for some people. They're afraid that worrying may make them mentally or physically ill. Or they may fear being unable to control their worry. But although worry is unpleasant and unproductive, it isn't dangerous – and you can learn to control it.

> *although worry is unpleasant and unproductive, it isn't dangerous – and you can learn to control it.*

- **Use worry periods.** A technique often recommended by psychologists is to save up your worrying for a daily twenty-minute 'worry period'. If you find yourself worrying outside your worry period, write down what's bugging you and then save it for later. Twenty minutes a day of worrying is plenty!

- **Don't fight your worries; let them go.** Simply watch the worry come into your mind, acknowledge it, but don't let it distract you. Stay as calm as you can, focus on what you're doing and not what you're thinking, and watch your worry recede into the distance.

- **Accept uncertainty.** No matter how much we worry, we can't know for sure what's in store for us. So don't dwell on hypothetical future problems; instead, focus on the positive things in your life right now. If you're finding it tough to think of those positives, try the exercises on pp. 70–6.

- **Have more fun!** When are you most likely to worry? Perhaps you tend to be anxious the night before going back to work after the weekend. Maybe you find yourself worrying when you first wake up. Try to identify the times when you're vulnerable to worry, and make sure you have an enjoyable activity lined up instead.

  For example, rather than spending your Sunday evenings fretting about work, make a regular date to see friends. If worry strikes first thing in the morning, reserve that time for a run or a meditation session (see Chapter 7 for more on meditation).

- **Learn from the people around you.** If you're having a tough time with worry, ask your trusted friends and family how they cope. They'll probably have some useful advice. And talking things over is an excellent way to get some perspective on your problems.

PROBLEM-SOLVING

When we worry we focus on the consequences of something bad happening. Psychologists call it 'what if?' thinking: 'What if I say something embarrassing?'; 'What if I miss my train?'; 'What if my friend had an accident?'

These thoughts can spiral out of control: this is known as *catastrophizing*. For example, imagine your friend's birthday is coming up next week and you're not sure what gift to buy. If you're a worrier, your thoughts might run like this:

- What if I buy something he doesn't like? He'll think less of me.

- What if he thinks less of me? He won't want to spend time with me.

- What if he doesn't want to spend time with me? He'll tell all our friends and they'll feel the same way.

- What if my other friends feel the same way? I'll be all alone.

- What if I'm all alone? I won't be able to cope.

So a worry about a birthday present has ended up with us friendless and isolated! This is pretty far-fetched, of course, but actually it's a good illustration of the way worry works. We spend a lot of time worrying about things that are very unlikely to happen. We don't take a balanced view of the situation: instead we focus on the negative. As you've probably discovered, worry can take you to some very gloomy, and very implausible places.

Life will throw you the occasional curve ball, for sure. But you'll cope. Instead of treating these challenges as catastrophes in waiting, opt to see them as problems to be solved. Change your perspective; from the negative to the positive, from passive to active.

> *Change your perspective; from the*
> *negative to the positive,*
> *from passive to active.*

Problem-solving is all about taking a logical approach to dealing with issues. And because it's logical, there's no mystery, no special trick. We can all learn how to do it. So think of a problem that's worrying you at the moment, and follow the steps below. Make sure you write down your answers.

1   Define the problem as specifically as you can.

2   Think of a range of possible solutions. What has worked for you in the past? Consider asking someone you trust for advice. What would you suggest that someone else with the same problem might do?

3   Weigh up the pros and cons of each possible solution.

4   Choose the solution you think is best and decide how you're going to carry it out. Try to guess what problems you might face and how you're going to deal with them.

5   Try out the solution you've chosen and then have a think about how well it's worked. If things haven't gone to plan, try the next solution.

I am not afraid of storms for I am learning how to sail my ship.
LOUISA MAY ALCOTT

BE COMFORTABLE WITH YOUR CHOICES

Here are two contrasting approaches to organising a weekend away at the seaside.

Chris pores over newspaper travel supplements, consults with friends and spends hours surfing the web, searching for deals on a hotel room and rail fare. Chris changes his mind constantly. Just when he thinks he's chosen a hotel, for example, he'll come across a negative review on the web. Just when he's about to book his train ticket, he wonders whether it would be cheaper if he went to a different resort. When he does make a decision, he is plagued by doubts. Even while he's away, he can't help wondering whether the hotel down the road would have been a better choice.

Megan has always liked Brighton, so she decides to head there. A friend mentions a cheap deal at a chain hotel. Although the reviews on the web are mixed, Megan sees this is true of two other hotels she checks. Besides, she tells herself, it's right on the beach, the price is good, and it's only for a couple of nights. She looks online for her train tickets, quickly finds what she feels is the best deal, and books. She can't wait for the weekend.

Life is full of decisions, from the trivial (Which pair of jeans should I buy? What colour should we paint the kitchen?) to the momentous (Which career should I train for? Should I move in with my partner?).

We tend to assume that our decisions can influence our level of happiness – and sometimes, of course, they do. But it's arguable that far more important for our contentment is our *attitude* towards those decisions.

Chris, for example, is what psychologists call a 'maximiser'. Before taking a decision, he carefully researches and weighs up the options. He agonises over every detail. But he's rarely happy with his decision; instead, he worries that he could have done better.

Megan, on the other hand, is a 'satisficer'. Instead of hours of deliberation, she is comfortable with the first option that appeals to her. Once she's made a decision, she seldom gives it another thought.

If you find decision-making difficult, aim to become more of a satisficer. To do this, aim to narrow your options down fast and then set a time limit for your decision. It often helps if you tell other people that you'll have made up your mind by a particular point. Look back at your previous decisions: wouldn't they have been just as good if they'd been made in half the time? Trust your judgement, enjoy your choices, and don't look back.

COPING WITH NEGATIVE THOUGHTS

The average person has more than 4000 thoughts each day, and some of them are usually negative. But it's how we respond to these thoughts that determines how problematic we find them.

When we're feeling down or anxious or stressed it's easy to take these negative thoughts at face value. But we need to treat them with caution. You can help yourself react in the right way by following these guidelines, which have been well-tested in clinical trials:

- **Don't treat thoughts as though they were facts.** Most of our thoughts are anything but reasoned and logical. Generally they're just a snap reaction to what we see or feel. Imagine for instance that a colleague passes you in the corridor without saying hello. If you're feeling a bit low, you might worry that they're deliberately ignoring you. But this reaction probably reveals far more about your own emotions than it does about your colleague's.

- **Think of the evidence for and against the thought.** What grounds do you have for believing that your colleague has ignored you? What evidence is there to the contrary?

- **Think of alternative explanations.** There are almost always several potential reasons for any event – perhaps your colleague is worried about an important meeting or has had a row with their partner; perhaps they've simply forgotten their glasses: you just have to take the time to think those reasons through.

● **Test out your explanations.** There's no better way to find out whether your assumptions are correct. If you're really worried that you've offended your colleague in some way, invite them to join you for lunch. You'll soon discover whether there are any grounds for your worries.

● **Drop your safety behaviours.** When we're worried about something, we often adopt a range of strategies designed to prevent the event we're anxious about from happening. Psychologists call these strategies 'safety behaviours'.

Safety behaviours may seem to be saving us from trouble, but in fact they keep our anxieties alive. This is because we assume our safety behaviours are the reason why nothing bad has occurred. We don't realise that actually there's no cause for concern.

So don't avoid your colleague until they forget whatever it is you fear you may have done to upset them. That would be a safety behaviour. Treat them just as you would normally. Don't let your worries fester: put them to the test.

● **Keep an open mind.** Most people want certainty most of the time, but we have to accept that there are some things we'll never know for sure. You can't be 100 per cent certain about what was going on in your colleague's head (though you can make a reasoned judgement). Think through the probabilities and then let the matter go.

Our greatest glory is not in never falling, but in rising every time we fall. CONFUCIUS (551–479 BC)

FROM SELF-CRITICISM TO SELF-COMPASSION

It's a curious thing: many of us are far more critical of ourselves than we are of other people. We say things about ourselves that we'd never dream of saying about anyone else. We give other people the benefit of the doubt but, where our own behaviour is concerned, quickly become angry or upset or disappointed. Again and again we jump to the same old conclusions: we're unattractive, we're stupid, we're fat, we're lazy, we're this, we're that...

This fault-finding, of course, often bears no relation to reality. In fact, it's remarkable how these negative attitudes persist despite all evidence to the contrary. The singer Duffy, for instance, has sold millions of albums worldwide and won Grammy and Brit awards for her work. But even after such phenomenal success, Duffy is still prone to self-criticism: 'I'm my own worst critic. Sometimes my own worst enemy. You'd have a hard time being tougher on me than I am on myself.'

If you recognise yourself in this description, now's the time to do something about it. Now's the time to reject self-criticism and replace it with *self-compassion*:

- Be kind to yourself, both in the way you think about yourself and in how you care for your body (see Chapter 2 for advice on improving your diet and sleep habits).

- Don't leap to judgement on yourself. Keep your mind and heart open.

- Accept and respect your needs and desires.

- Allow yourself to communicate those needs and desires to other people. You have a right to be heard.

- Celebrate your many achievements and forgive any occasional lapses.

- Fill your life with activities that make you happy (to find out how, see Chapter 4).

To help you build your self-compassion, try this exercise: write down five positive qualities you believe you possess. Perhaps, for example, you're generous, or loving, or friendly. Rate how strongly you believe each statement.

	POSITIVE QUALITY	RATING (0–100%)
1		
2		
3		
4		
5		

Now try to recall specific examples of these positive qualities. Close your eyes and visualise them as clearly as you can. Over the next week, try to notice these qualities in action. Take a few moments at the end of each day to write down the examples you've spotted.

> *You yourself, as much as anyone in the entire universe, deserve your love and affection.* THE BUDDHA

AVOID COMPARING YOURSELF TO OTHERS

Do you remember the phrase *Jante-lov*?

It's the Danish term we discussed in Chapter 1. It means: 'You're no better than anyone else.' It also implies that no one is better than you.

This can be a difficult message to remember if we're given to comparing ourselves to other people. Research has shown that frequent comparison with others can get us down, and lead to feelings of defeat. Take Paul, for example. He's in his early forties; lives in a large house in a pleasant suburb; enjoys a close and loving relationship with his wife; has four great children and many friends; and holds down a well-paid and stimulating job with a software company. You might think Paul has it made, but here's what he sees when he looks around him:

- I've got the oldest car of any of the managers at work.
- Ben's my age and he's so much fitter than me.
- Mark's kids are getting better results at school than mine.
- I love the way Beth and Joe have decorated their house, but ours seems tatty in comparison.
- Ben and Lisa are off to San Francisco this summer. Last year they were in Thailand. I never go anywhere interesting.
- Other people just look happier than I am.

Paul isn't untypical. If we're in the habit of comparing our lives to those of the people around us, it's easy to conclude that we're somehow inadequate.

Far better instead to:

- accept and value yourself
- celebrate the many positive aspects of your life
- recognise that, if things aren't perfect, that's normal and natural
- remember you don't know how the people you compare yourself to are *really* feeling
- resist the temptation to compare yourself to other people.

The trick, in other words, is to treat yourself with compassion.

> " *frequent comparison with others can get us down, and lead to feelings of defeat.* "

Of course, doing this in a society like ours that worships wealth, material possessions and celebrity can be a challenge. As we saw in Chapter 1, none of these things will guarantee us happiness. But a daily media diet of young, rich and beautiful celebrities, or the smiling folk in adverts, is enough to make anyone believe they have drawn life's short straw.

If you're prone to these kinds of worries, try changing the kind of newspapers and magazines you read, and the TV programmes you watch. For a week, put yourself on a celebrity and advert-free media diet. Notice any differences?

Everyone experiences negative thoughts and feelings from time to time, but you can prevent them dragging your mood downwards. There's so much you can do to take control – as we hope this chapter has demonstrated. But like all the practical suggestions in this book, don't take our word for it: try these techniques out. We believe you'll notice the benefits straight away.

Now let's turn to the strategies you can use to increase your *positive* thoughts.

CHAPTER 6
Increasing positive thoughts

Chapter 5 was all about learning to calm your negative thoughts. Now it's time to focus on the positive.

The activities in this chapter will help you appreciate the good things in your life now, and the good things you may not have been able to appreciate in the past. It'll then help you look forward to a happier future. Drawing on the findings of both CBT and the new science of positive psychology, we'll explain how to boost your positive thoughts, mental images, feelings and behaviours.

Even the way we use our body can affect the way we feel. For example, research has shown that nodding our head, in comparison with shaking it, can make us feel more positive about a previously neutral object! If we nod our head when learning a list of words, we're better at remembering the positive words; if we shake our head, we're more able to recall negative words. Other experiments have demonstrated that simply changing our facial expression, or posture, or hand and arm movements can influence our emotions.

What this shows is that we have much more power over our thoughts and feelings than we might imagine. We don't have to wait for happiness to suddenly appear in our lives; we can help generate it ourselves.

WHAT'S GOING RIGHT FOR ME RIGHT NOW?

This is a very simple exercise developed by one of the leading psychologists of happiness, Barbara Fredrickson. All you need to do is pause, look around you and ask yourself: *'what is going right for me right now?'* If you find it difficult to think of anything positive, try to keep going until you have at least one example.

Here's an ordinary day, ordinary life kind of example:

● Beautiful weather outside

● Feeling rested and healthy

● Got some work done this morning

● Cat dozing on a nearby chair

● Looking forward to a mid-morning cup of coffee!

There are two really nice things about this particular activity. First is the fact that spending just a few moments focusing on the positive things in your current situation boosts your mood. Secondly, identifying what's good in your life allows you to seek more of it. For example, though there's not much we can do about the weather, we can note our satisfaction at a productive morning's work and aim to reproduce that feeling as often as possible.

SAVOURING

Think of increasing your happiness as a skill: a set of strategies and techniques everyone can learn. One of the key components of that skill is the ability to recognise and *savour* the good things in life, no matter how small. By savouring we mean taking the time to notice, and delight in, an experience – to really kick back and bask in the pleasure of the moment, and to try to make that pleasure *last*.

> *Living in the moment means letting go of the past and not waiting for the future. It means living your life consciously, aware that each moment you breathe is a gift.* OPRAH WINFREY

If you've completed the 'What's going right for me right now' exercise on the previous page, you've already sampled the pleasures of savouring. You've applied a temporary brake to the passing of time. You've created a space in which you can look around and remind yourself of some of the pleasing features of your life. If we don't learn to savour, it's easy to take those features for granted or to miss them entirely.

> *remind yourself of some of the pleasing features of your life. If we don't learn to savour, it's easy to take those features for granted.*

The 'What's going right for me right now?' exercise helps you to savour the present moment. There are other, very simple ways of doing this, too. For example, we can take a little time each day to really focus on what we're doing and how we're feeling. Give it a go when, for instance, you next eat a piece of fruit; spend time with friends; finish a piece of work you're pleased with; or simply breathe the fresh air outside.

Try to take in every detail of the moment; revel in your enjoyment. What are your senses telling you? Focus on the precise taste of the fruit; feel the breeze play across your face; listen intently to your friends' voices. Give yourself up to the moment; aim to inhabit it with your whole spirit.

Savouring isn't merely something we can do in the present. We can savour the future and the past too. Whether it's a holiday you've just booked, a meal you're cooking for friends, a walk in the countryside, a massage, or a trip to buy new clothes, spend a few minutes each day actively looking forward to these treats. Allow yourself the luxury of a daydream, especially if you're feeling low: thinking about future fun is sure to pick you up.

Even when the event you've looked forward to is over, it can still be a great source of pleasure. Make the effort to remember what happened and relish every little detail. Take photos. Relive the moment by reminiscing with friends. Perhaps write a brief note of what happened and, in particular, how much happiness it gave you.

If you can savour an experience beforehand, while it's happening, and afterwards, think how far you're making that pleasure go!

Happy memories make a brilliant pick-me-up. A nice idea suggested by the psychologist Sonia Lyubomirsky is to create a 'savouring album'. Fill it with photos and other mementoes of all that is dearest to you in life – perhaps your friends, partner, children, pet, home, or souvenirs from a special holiday. Don't bury the album away in a drawer; keep it somewhere accessible. Perhaps, as Lyubomirsky does, take it with you when you travel. That way, it'll always be on hand when you need a lift.

GRATITUDE

> *I would maintain that thanks are the highest form of thought; and that gratitude is happiness doubled by wonder.* G.K. CHESTERTON

You've probably seen one of those famous 'Love is...' cartoon strips. Well, if we were creating a version on the subject of happiness it might read something like this:

Happiness is... always being thankful.

This is because one of the hallmarks of happy people is a deeply engrained sense of gratitude – to other people, for sure, but more broadly to life itself.

Perhaps, for example, you can remember waking up on a beautiful summer's day. It was a Saturday. You felt rested and healthy. The week's hassles and stresses had vanished overnight. Ahead of you was a day of relaxation and fun – perhaps a treat you'd been looking forward to for ages, or simply a quiet day pottering contentedly around the house. And, as you lay there in bed, feeling the sun warming your body, you thought to yourself: *How lucky I am to be alive!*

Or perhaps you can recall a time when you were suffering from flu. You struggled in to work, but by mid-morning you were feeling awful. Not only did your manager send you home, she took the time to drive you there herself. Over the next few days, friends brought you medicines and food and books and magazines. Each evening someone would phone to see how you were. You were so grateful for their efforts and thankful to have such good friends.

This is gratitude in action. We recognise, celebrate and treasure the many positive aspects to our life. And it feels great.

Bliss was it in that dawn to be alive. WILLIAM WORDSWORTH

For some people, gratitude seems to come naturally. But if you're not among them, don't worry: gratitude can be learned.

One very effective technique is simply to write down, every night for two weeks, five things in your life for which you are grateful. Those things can be as minor, or as important, as you like. For example:

- Really enjoyable lunch with colleagues at work.

- My cold has disappeared! I'm back on form now.

- Feel so lucky to have met my partner.

- Dad is recovering really well from his operation.

- Favourite programme on TV this evening!

At the end of those two weeks, how has your mood improved?

If you're finding this activity helpful – and lots of people do – consider making it a part of your routine. Some people prefer to complete their gratitude log once or twice a week. Experiment, and go with what works best for you, but try to stick to a regular time – for example, writing every Monday night. That way, there's less chance of it being crowded out of your schedule by other commitments.

Think too about taking your gratitude out into the world and directly thanking the people who contribute – in however small a way – to your happiness.

This isn't just good manners; it's about increasing the sum total of happiness in the world. And to do that, your gratitude has to be heartfelt. Doesn't it feel good when someone thanks you? Isn't it even better when they smile as well? The glow it transmits can last all day.

So, if someone moves aside to help you make your way down the bus, thank them. If your neighbour takes in a parcel while you're out, thank them. And find a moment to thank those closest to you simply for being there. That may seem a bit too sentimental, but try it. You – and the people you thank – will feel all the better for it.

RECORDING THE POSITIVES

To savour the good things in life, it stands to reason that we have to be able to spot them. If we can't see the positives, we can't celebrate them.

> *If we can't see the positives, we can't celebrate them.*

But noticing the good stuff isn't always easy, particularly on those days when we're feeling down. If you're finding it difficult at the moment, this exercise will help.

What we want you to do is keep a diary *for seven days* of the positive things you do or that happen to you. It needn't be very time-consuming; all you have to do is make a brief note of the positive event and how it made you feel at the time. Look for the little details: perhaps a colleague helped you with a task, you had a pleasant walk home in the sunshine, or you enjoyed a great movie.

Here's a format you could use:

DAY	POSITIVE THING	HOW DO YOU FEEL?

And here's an excerpt from a diary compiled by Sam, a thirty-six-year-old sales executive:

DAY	POSITIVE THING	HOW DO YOU FEEL?
Monday	Listened to my MP3 player on the train in to work.	Completely absorbed in the music; can't get enough of that new album.
	Bought a latte from the canteen.	Love my cup of coffee in the morning.
	Complimentary email from client.	Proud. Gave me a lift just when I needed it.
	Good chat with Chris, Rob and Louise over lunch. Lots of laughter.	Left the canteen with a smile on my face. Happy to have such good mates at work.
	Phone call from Allie; she's got tickets for the theatre next weekend – wanted to know if I could come.	Excited, and pleased to have been asked.

DAY	POSITIVE THING	HOW DO YOU FEEL?
	Afternoon coffee. Treated myself to a piece of carrot cake and ate it at a table in the canteen, rather than at my desk.	Cake delicious. Pepped me up for the remainder of the afternoon. And great to have ten minutes' break.
	Finished writing monthly report.	Relieved.
	Gorgeous summer evening as I walked to the train station. Sky a deep, cloudless blue.	Optimistic.
	Long soak in the bath.	Relaxed.
	Curled up in bed with the thriller Louise lent me.	Totally gripped! Kept meaning to turn off the light, but couldn't resist another chapter.

At the end of the seven days, make yourself a cup of tea, find somewhere quiet, and spend some time looking back over your diary. We think you'll be pleasantly surprised at just how many nice things have occurred during the week, and at how often you've experienced a little frisson of enjoyment.

You'll find too that keeping the diary has honed your pleasure-spotting skills. The next time something positive occurs – and you won't have to wait long – you'll notice it straight away.

OPTIMISM

Everything I've done I've done with enthusiasm and
passion. Everything I turn up to, I think I'm going to enjoy.
KEVIN KEEGAN

Many people think that optimism is something you're born with: you either have it or you don't. It's true that optimism comes easier to some people than others, but optimism is a style of thinking – and styles of thinking can be learned.

This is great news. Almost by definition, when you think more optimistically you'll feel more confident, more relaxed, and happier all round. But there are other advantages. For example, optimism helps us achieve our goals in life: we're much more likely to keep going if we think we'll be successful in the end. It helps us cope when times are tough. And at least two major research studies suggest that it can help us live longer too.

> *when you think more optimistically*
> *you'll feel more confident, more relaxed,*
> *and happier all round.*

Optimism is all about our expectations for the future. If we're optimistic, we expect that future to turn out well – both the big stuff (for example, living a long, happy and healthy life) and the comparatively insignificant (like whether the new recipe you're trying out tonight will taste as good as it looks in the book).

At the heart of the optimistic (or pessimistic) style of thinking is a distinctive way of explaining negative and positive events, particularly in situations where the true cause isn't obvious.

Putting it very simply, when something good happens to an optimist, they tend to assume it's down to them. Perhaps it's something they did, or a consequence of the way they are. Moreover, not only does the optimist think this particular good thing is likely to happen again, they're confident that lots more good things will come their way in the future.

How does an optimist react to negative events? Their instinct is to see them as one-offs – things may have gone wrong on this occasion, but next time will be better. They may feel that it's not their fault, but if they do decide they're to blame they won't beat themselves up about it. Instead they'll be certain they won't make the same error again.

A pessimist, on the other hand, is likely to react in exactly the opposite fashion. A positive event is a fluke that has nothing to do with them. A negative event is their fault, and an indication of what lies ahead in the future.

To take an example, let's imagine that an optimist and a pessimist sit a maths test. They both achieve great marks. The optimist will believe their success is a result of intelligence, and be confident that they'll fare well in other exams. The pessimist, however, will conclude that they just got lucky or scraped through because they worked much harder than everyone else. Rather than gaining confidence from their performance, they'll fear the worst for future tests.

Some days later, our optimist and pessimist take a history test. Both score poorly. The optimist will conclude that the questions were misleading, or their answers misunderstood, or that their low mark is the result of chronic hayfever. They'll be sure that the next time they take a history test they'll do much better. The pessimist, however, will see the result as proof of how poor they are at exams, and will doubt that they'll ever improve.

Take a moment to reflect on your own experience. Which approach do you most often use to make sense of the things that happen to you: the pessimistic or the optimistic? If it's the pessimistic, you're almost certainly too hard on yourself when events don't go well and you don't give yourself enough credit when good things happen. Setbacks seem like portents of the future and positive events like flukes.

If you're prone to pessimism, take heart from the fact that you can change your typical thinking style. You can learn optimism. And when you do you'll notice the positive effect on your mood.

A quick guide to developing the inner optimist

To become more optimistic, keep a close eye on the way you explain events. Make a conscious effort to adopt an optimistic style of thinking. With practice, it'll develop into second nature. If you spot a pessimistic thought, challenge it using the techniques on pp. 62–3.

Here's another exercise to boost your optimism. This one was developed by the psychologist Laura King and it involves imagining your 'best possible future self'. Research has demonstrated that just carrying out this exercise alone produces significant increases in optimism.

For a fortnight, spend five minutes each day writing about how you see yourself a few years from now *when all your hopes have been realised*. You might, for instance, have the job you've always dreamed of. You might be living in your favourite city. You might be happily married with a strong network of close friends nearby.

Simply committing your hopes to paper is likely to make you feel more optimistic about the future. But you can also use the exercise to help turn those dreams into reality.

Once you've identified where you'd like to be in a few years' time, think about the steps you'll need to take to get there. You already have your long-term target, now add the short- and medium-term goals that will help you reach that objective.

Every few months revisit your 'best possible self' document. It'll help you check that you're still on course to meet your goals, and provide brilliant motivation if you find yourself flagging. You can remind yourself: *this* is where I'm going. This is worth working for. (Of course, if your priorities have changed, by all means amend what you've written.)

This technique of imagining future success can be used in all sorts of situations. Perhaps you have an interview for a job coming up. Maybe you've agreed to give a speech at a friend's wedding. Or perhaps you need to have a difficult conversation with someone. Whatever the upcoming challenge, the trick is to *visualise* it turning out well. Include as much detail as possible, and rehearse your part as often as you can.

Visualisation is a staple of sports psychology. Many, many world champions have used it to help them achieve their goals. And it can work for you too.

> *The very least you can do in your life is to figure out what you hope for. And the most you can do is live inside that hope. Not admire it from a distance but live right in it, under its roof.* BARBARA KINGSOLVER

As with all habits, changing from a pessimistic to an optimistic viewpoint can take a bit of time. If you usually point out the downsides to a situation, or have got used to balancing out someone you feel is too naively positive, you might find it tricky at first to alter your instinctive reactions. The trick is to:

- become aware of those pessimistic reactions
- avoid automatically accepting them; instead, pause, recognise what they are and challenge them: ask yourself what the evidence is for and against
- appreciate that there are other ways of looking at the situation
- consciously replace them with positive thoughts.

In time, you'll find that optimism becomes your default setting.

SOUNDS AND MUSIC

Fans of The Simpsons may remember the episode in which Homer is misinformed that he has only twenty-four hours to live. As he listens to Lisa playing a melancholy tune on her saxophone, he breaks down in tears. This, you might think, is hardly surprising given his predicament.

Yet, as Lisa rapidly switches to an upbeat number, Homer's mood is miraculously transformed. Indeed, he is soon dancing his way around Lisa's bedroom and out the door. As he departs, we hear his joyful singing: 'Oh, I want to be in that rumba when the saints go over there!'

It's a touching scene – and one that demonstrates the enormously powerful effect music can have on our emotions. Psychologists have done a lot of research in this area and the evidence is clear: relaxing music calms us; happy music cheers us up.

What this means in practice is that you can increase your well-being by choosing the right kind of music. If that seems too good to be true, we urge you to put it to the test!

Try putting together a compilation CD for those times when you need a lift. (If you've ever fancied choosing your Desert Island discs, you should definitely enjoy this exercise.) In fact, you might want to have one selection to get you feeling up and bouncy, and another to help you chill out at the end of a tiring day.

When the mental health charity Mind carried out a survey, these were the top three songs for happiness:

- 'Let Me Entertain You' – Robbie Williams
- 'Walking on Sunshine' – Katrina and the Waves
- 'Shiny Happy People' – REM

And these were rated best for relaxation:

- 'Thank You' – Dido
- 'Bridge Over Troubled Waters' – Simon and Garfunkel
- 'Porcelain' – Moby

Of course, music isn't the only type of sound that can increase our well-being. Relaxation CDs are enormously popular and tend to feature sounds from the natural world: for example, surf rolling onto a beach, the dawn chorus, a running stream, the gentle pattering of rain in a forest, whale song. You may find your public library has something suitable, or perhaps you can borrow a CD from a friend, and there are plenty now on YouTube. Give it a try and see whether it works for you too.

Remember also that *making* music is a terrific way of increasing well-being. If you used to play an instrument or sing, why not take it up again? A local band, choir or orchestra is sure to want you!

If you haven't played or sung before, why not start now? You don't need to be proficient to derive pleasure from music-making. Even the rawest novice will experience a huge amount of fun and a morale-boosting sense of achievement as they gradually improve. We speak from personal experience...

Remember the four components of happiness we discussed in Chapter 1? Making music is a perfect means to experience engagement or flow, and if you're doing it with other people, a great way to build friendships.

If structured music-making isn't your thing, there's always the joy of singing for your own pleasure. So, whether you sing in the shower or along to favourite songs on the radio or CD player, open those lungs and let it out!

HUMOUR

'Laughter, by definition, is healthy,' wrote the South African novelist Doris Lessing. She was absolutely right. In fact, scientists have suggested that a sense of humour is one of the major influences on longevity.

But whether or not laughter helps us live longer isn't our primary concern. What we're after is a boost to our mood, an increase in positivity – and laughter definitely ticks that box. Think of your own experience – don't you feel better after sharing a joke with friends or watching a funny movie?

So the objective of this particular exercise is simple: we want you to spend more time laughing, chuckling and giggling. If you can achieve that by hanging out with friends, so much the better. But don't forget that you have at your disposal a huge range of funny films, books and TV and radio programmes – all of them carefully crafted to make you smile.

Doubtless you have your own favourites, but if you fancy something new ask your friends for suggestions.

I am thankful for laughter, except when milk comes out of my nose. WOODY ALLEN

SMILE, SMILE, SMILE!

The human brain is an extraordinarily complex organ. It's far more powerful and sophisticated than any computer, for instance. And yet the brain can be fooled by something as simple as a smile.

Many experiments have demonstrated that we can produce an emotion in ourselves just by adopting the appropriate facial expression. Pretend to frown, for example, and your mood will dip. Feign a smile, on the other hand, and you'll actually feel happier.

Try it out for a day. Every couple of hours, and whether you feel like it or not, spend a few minutes smiling. To help you, think of a happy memory, a time when you had the giggles, or a favourite joke. And yes, this might feel a bit weird to start with, but just try it and hang in there.

Aside from a positive effect on your own mood, one of the big changes you may notice is the behaviour of other people. We're hard-wired from birth to respond positively to another person's smile. Even as adults, we are drawn to the people who are fun to be around. If someone smiles when they see you, don't you light up inside?

When you smile more often, you'll find that your interactions with other people change accordingly. Because you project feelings of warmth, friendliness and approachability, you'll be treated in kind. Which means that you won't be the only person doing more smiling!

In the next chapter you'll find more strategies to boost your positive thoughts and feelings. This time the focus is on relaxation, meditation and a new, but already hugely popular, psychological technique for increasing well-being: mindfulness. So read on and prepare to chill out!

> *When you arise in the morning, think of what a precious privilege it is to be alive – to breathe, to think, to enjoy, to love.* MARCUS AURELIUS (121–180 AD), ROMAN EMPEROR

CHAPTER 7

Relaxing your body and mind

How do you like to relax? Assuming that you do relax somehow, of course... Do you sleep? Run? Socialise? Do something creative? Get outdoors?

We all have our favourite ways to unwind. However, it can be a bit hit and miss. What works for one person may be less effective for someone else. One survey revealed that some people relax by surfing the internet or making lists of things to do – the rest of us might find both these things have the opposite effect! And an activity that relaxes us one day may not be so effective on another.

So, in this chapter we focus on techniques that are specifically designed – and scientifically proven – to produce deep relaxation of both body and mind, no matter how you're feeling on a given day. Over the coming weeks, aim to give them all a try. You may find some suit you more than others, which is absolutely fine. Stick with the ones that are most effective for you.

And that phrase 'sticking with it' is important. To really experience the benefit that these techniques can bring, you need to make them a regular part of your life. A huge time commitment isn't necessary – fifteen to twenty minutes a day will do it – but it's best to perform your chosen activity every day.

> *To really experience the benefit that these techniques can bring, you need to make them a regular part of your life.*

Like so many things in life, developing a relaxation routine is often more enjoyable when we do it in company. We're also more likely to persist with an activity when we're part of a group. So it's a good idea to investigate classes and clubs in your area. Activities like meditation and yoga are hugely popular, which means there's a good chance you'll find something suitable nearby.

Remember too that there's a mass of information out there to help you get the most from your relaxation activity. Whether it's yoga, mindfulness, or some other form of relaxation technique, you'll find lots of useful books, audio CDs and websites on the topic.

PROGRESSIVE MUSCLE RELAXATION

An anxious mind cannot exist in a relaxed body.
EDMUND JACOBSON

When we're feeling stressed, the restless tension of our thoughts is mirrored in our body. Our muscles tighten, our heart rate increases and our breathing becomes faster and shallower.

To calm this physical tension, the US doctor Edmund Jacobson (1888–1983) developed a technique called *progressive muscle relaxation*. The idea is that each group of muscles in your body is tensed and released in turn. Once you've tensed the muscle consciously, it's much easier to then consciously relax it. You can follow the order of muscles outlined here, or vary the pattern if you prefer. The key point is to gradually progress around your body and to include a good range of the major muscles.

Choose a time and place when you know you won't be disturbed. Make yourself comfortable. Take off your shoes; loosen any tight clothing. Sit in a chair or, if you're confident you won't fall asleep, lie down on the floor, or on a bed or sofa. Close your eyes.

For a minute or so, concentrate on breathing deeply and slowly. Feel your body begin to relax.

Clench both fists as tightly as you can. Count to ten and then release. Enjoy the relaxation of your muscles for approximately twenty seconds, then move on to the next exercise.

Tense the muscles in your neck and shoulders by lifting your shoulders up to your ears. Again, hold for ten seconds and then relax for twenty seconds.

Moving on to the muscles in your face, press your teeth together as firmly as you can. At the same time, keep your eyelids tightly closed. Hold for ten seconds and relax for the standard twenty seconds.

Now focus on your chest. Take a deep breath and, after counting to ten, exhale gently.

Clench your stomach muscles, hold for a count of ten, and then release.

Now it's time to work on your feet and legs. Press down with your legs then flex your toes upwards to work your calf muscles. Finally, pull your toes downwards to tense the muscles in your feet. For all three manoeuvres, hold for ten seconds and then release for twenty seconds.

When you've completed this cycle of exercises, let yourself rest. Notice how the tension has left your body. Savour the feeling of deep relaxation that has taken its place. Enjoy the steady rhythm of your breathing. If you detect any tightness in your body, flex the muscles in question and then release.

Aim to spend about ten minutes each day on progressive muscle relaxation. Find a convenient time – perhaps first thing in the morning or when you arrive home from work – and make it a regular date.

A VISUALISATION EXERCISE

Here's a very quick but effective relaxation exercise that's designed to conjure up in your mind a soothing, pleasing image. It's a great technique to have up your sleeve, especially when you're feeling stressed or anxious.

Start by finding a quiet and comfortable place where you won't be disturbed. Turn off your mobile! You might want to play some calming music in the background.

Now close your eyes and imagine your favourite, most relaxing place. Perhaps it's an idyllic beach, a deserted meadow by a trickling stream, or a spectacular mountainside.

Imagine how it would feel for you to be there right now. Focus on the colours, the scenery, the sounds and the smells. Allow yourself to drift into this wonderfully relaxing scene.

Aim to spend five minutes on this exercise, once or twice a day.

YOGA

People have been using yoga to relax for centuries, and its effectiveness is increasingly backed up by clinical trials.

You can try out yoga using one of the dozens of books, CDs and DVDs that are available, but to really get the most from it, we recommend you join a class. This might seem a bit daunting, but yoga is a wonderfully non-competitive activity. Rather than aiming to outdo you, you'll find that the other members of your class are friendly and supportive. No one, bar the teacher, is going to be paying any attention to how you're getting on with the exercises: they'll be absorbed in their own efforts. Classes are run for all levels of experience and mobility, and for both men and women.

MINDFULNESS

One of the most popular new relaxation techniques is called *mindfulness*. It's essentially a blend of modern Western psychology and ancient Buddhist beliefs and practices, though you don't have to be spiritually inclined to practise it successfully. There's increasing scientific evidence to suggest that mindfulness is a powerful tool to calm negative thoughts and boost well-being.

> *mindfulness is a powerful tool to calm
> negative thoughts and boost well-being.*

Mindfulness focuses on living in the present, without worrying about the past or future, and seeing our thoughts as passing mental events, rather than reflections of truth or reality.

Here's how mindfulness is described by four of its pioneers: Mark Williams, John Teasdale, Zindel Segal and Jon Kabat-Zinn:

> Mindfulness is the awareness that arises from paying attention on purpose, in the present moment, non-judgementally, to things as they are. Mindfulness is not paying more attention but paying attention differently and more wisely – with the whole mind and heart, using the full resources of the body and its sense.

THE RAISIN MEDITATION

The capacity for delight is the gift of paying attention.
JULIA CAMERON

To enjoy a taste of mindfulness, try the following brief exercise. All you need is five minutes to yourself and a few raisins. If you don't like raisins, feel free to use something else – perhaps a piece of fruit, or a biscuit, or a square of chocolate. Your aim is to experience that item of food as fully as you possibly can.

Begin by picking up a raisin. For about twenty seconds, concentrate on how it *feels* in your hand; its texture and weight, the sensations it produces in contact with your skin.

Then focus on how the raisin *looks*. Try to take in every detail, as if you were looking at a rare and precious jewel. Again, spend about twenty seconds on this stage (and on the others that follow).

Hold the raisin to your nose. How does it *smell*? Breathe deeply; savour the raisin's scent.

Next, carefully place the raisin *on your tongue*. Let it rest there while you notice exactly how it feels. Then gently examine the raisin with your tongue.

Begin to *chew* the raisin. Do it slowly, and focus your attention on the taste and texture. How does your mouth feel? How would you describe this experience to someone who had never tasted a raisin?

When you're ready, gradually *swallow* the raisin. Again, try to register every last detail of the process. Concentrate as if you were performing the most intricate manoeuvre rather than simply swallowing some dried fruit.

Lastly, think about how it feels now that you've swallowed the raisin. Can you still taste it? Do you detect its scent? What sensations do you notice in your mouth and teeth?

What did you make of the experience as a whole? Did you notice a new intensity to the relatively humdrum act of eating a raisin? Did you feel your awareness blossom into life? This intensity, this awareness, is mindfulness in action.

The best way to develop mindfulness is through regular, daily meditation. The rest of this chapter presents a number of meditations for you to try, but you don't need to limit yourself to these more formal exercises – you can practise mindful meditation in almost any situation. In particular, it's a great way of freshening up dull chores and mundane activities, whether it's walking to work, doing the ironing, or washing the dishes. As the Buddhist monk, Thich Nhat Hanh, has commented:

> While washing the dishes one should only be washing the dishes, which means one should be completely aware of the fact that one is washing the dishes. At first glance, that might seem a little silly. Why put so much stress on a simple thing? But that's precisely the point. The fact that I am standing there and washing these bowls is a wondrous reality. I am completely myself, following my breath, conscious of my presence, and conscious of my thoughts and actions. There's no way I can be tossed around mindlessly like a bottle slapped here and there on the waves.

A BREATHING MEDITATION

This is a great meditation for beginners – and for everyone else too. You have just one aim: to concentrate on your breathing.

Begin by making yourself comfortable in your meditation position. The classic meditating pose is seated on the floor or on a cushion with your legs crossed. Of course, that isn't comfortable for everyone – for example, those of us with bad backs!

What you're after is a position that you can maintain for ten or twenty minutes without discomfort. If you're unhappy with your position it'll only distract you from your meditation. Ideally, your back will be straight and your posture upright.

If sitting on your bottom on the floor isn't right for you, try a firm, straight-backed chair. Kneeling can be good too, as long as your knees are up to it. Position a cushion between your bottom and your feet.

If sitting isn't possible for you, don't worry, you can meditate standing up, walking, or lying down. As ever, it's good to experiment and discover the position that suits you best.

Wear loose, comfortable clothing and, as with all the relaxation exercises in this chapter, it's crucial that you aren't disturbed. Trying to meditate while your children yell for attention, or your housemate sings along to the radio, or the cat miaows for food is taking optimism a step too far! So find that secluded spot and make the next ten minutes all your own.

When you're ready to begin, close your eyes and direct your attention to the rise and fall of your breathing. Observe how your body behaves when you inhale and exhale: how your abdomen gradually rises and falls; the sensation in your nostrils; the feeling in your lungs and chest.

Notice the rhythm of your breathing. Let your mind focus on the cycle of inhalation and exhalation. The breath in and the breath out.

You may find that your breathing becomes deeper and more regular during the meditation. If that happens, great; if it doesn't, well that's fine too. Just let your breathing happen naturally. There's no need to alter it in any way.

Almost certainly you'll find that your mind wanders during the meditation. You might, for example, suddenly wonder what you're going to cook for supper tonight, or remember a remark someone made to you. Perhaps you'll worry that these interruptions mean you're not meditating 'correctly'.

Don't become disheartened if thoughts and feelings pop into your mind like this. It's absolutely normal, even for experienced meditators. Simply return your attention to your breathing – if necessary, over and over again.

Keep going with the meditation for about ten minutes.

THE BODY SCAN MEDITATION

In this meditation we're going to direct our attention to the various parts of our body. It's a meditative tour from head to toe – or rather from toe to head!

As with all meditations, your first task is to make yourself comfortable. For this exercise it's best to be lying down. That could be on your bed, on a sofa, or even the floor if that's what you prefer.

Ensure you won't be interrupted. This is another great reason to develop a meditation routine. By meditating at the same time each day – and in the same place – not only does it become a habit for you, the other people in your life understand that those twenty or thirty minutes are your private, personal time. This saves you having to explain for the umpteenth time that you don't want a cup of tea right now; you can't answer the phone when it rings; and you definitely aren't free to cook dinner/tidy up/unload the washing machine!

Begin the meditation by directing your attention to your body as a whole. Tune in to the sensations in those parts of your body that touch the surface you're lying on – for example, the back of your head, your shoulders, buttocks, legs, heels. Feel the tension in your muscles and limbs ebb away.

Now turn your attention to your toes and feet. How do they feel? If you don't sense anything much, don't worry. If you notice aches and pains, don't be concerned. *What* you feel isn't important; your objective is simply to become aware of a particular area of your body.

In due course let your attention begin its travels around your body. Gradually move from your feet and toes to your ankles, then your calves, thighs, hips, genitals, stomach, chest, lungs, arms and hands. After your hands, switch your awareness to your neck, face and head. Spend as long as you like on each part of your body, though aim for a minimum of 15–20 seconds.

At each point in your journey, gently note the feeling in that part of your body. Don't try to analyse that feeling; don't try to change it. Simply let it fill your mind. If other thoughts pop up – and they often do – don't fight them. It's nothing to worry about. Merely direct your attention back to your body.

The meditation ends as it began. Turn your mind to your body as a whole. Again, don't analyse or judge or try to alter anything, simply rest in awareness. Allow yourself to be borne along by the full swell of sensation. Give yourself up to the moment. When you're ready, open your eyes, stretch and gently sit up.

> *We live in this crazy world, full of jobs, and we have to be there, be-be-be – it's a very demanding, taxing world. The result of meditating is watching your thoughts, detachment from your own precepts of what is right and wrong, things that frustrate you, that you can't grasp and want to grasp onto.* GOLDIE HAWN

COMPASSIONATE MEDITATION

> *Come out of the circle of time and into the circle of love.*
> RUMI (1207–73), PERSIAN POET

The objective of compassionate meditation is to develop your positive feelings for yourself, the people you know, and those you will never meet. For many people, maybe in particular the

British, and perhaps especially men, it's more difficult than a breathing or body scan meditation; openly expressing our emotions isn't something that comes naturally to lots of us. But do give this meditation a try. After all, no one else will know what you're thinking!

Imagine for a moment that you love yourself as deeply as you love your child or partner or best friend.

Now picture yourself experiencing heartfelt affection not simply for those closest to you, but for the nameless people you pass in the street and even for the mass of humanity you have never encountered.

If we could feel like this, wouldn't we experience a wonderful sense of well-being? Wouldn't our days be filled with pleasure, enjoyment and contentment? Wouldn't the world seem a much happier place than it sometimes does today? This vision is the driving force behind compassionate (or loving-kindness) meditation.

Begin the meditation by tuning in to the rhythm of your breathing and the sensations of your body.

When you're relaxed and ready, visualise a person whom you have loved deeply and who has loved you. Think back to the times you spent with them and how their love made you feel.

Try to recall a particular moment in as much detail as you can. Let yourself experience once again the emotions you felt then: the love, contentment and joy. In your mind, communicate your love to the person you have chosen. Allow the warmth of your affection to radiate out towards them.

Many people find it helpful during this meditation to express their love through words. You could say to yourself versions of traditional Buddhist phrases: 'May they be safe. May they be happy. May they be free from suffering. May they be peaceful.' Alternatively, choose something that is especially meaningful to you.

Now direct that love – and those compassionate words – towards yourself. If you find this difficult, awkward or embarrassing, keep going. It will become easier. Remember: you are entitled to your love. *You deserve your love.*

If your compassion does not include yourself, it is incomplete. BUDDHA

Then, in turn, bring to mind someone you know well and care for, a person you see occasionally but have no feelings for, and someone who has annoyed or upset you in the past. To each of these individuals, reach out with love and compassion. Feel the waves of your loving-kindness emanating from your heart. Bask in this warmth.

Finally, let your love embrace every living being on the planet. To help you do this try visualising the Earth and, while you do so, repeat your compassionate phrases. Enjoy your feelings of love. Savour the contentment they have inspired in you. Delight in these sensations for as long as you choose.

THE THREE-MINUTE BREATHING SPACE MEDITATION

In many ways this is the perfect meditation: all it requires is three minutes of your time. It was developed by Mark Williams, John Teasdale, Zindel Segal and Jon Kabat-Zinn, all of whom have made a huge contribution to the development of mindfulness techniques.

The meditation is structured in three parts. Your focus will move from your thoughts and feelings to your breathing, then finally to your whole body.

You can do this meditation sitting or standing (but preferably not lying down). Hold yourself upright, though make sure it's a position you can adopt comfortably for the duration of the meditation.

For the first minute or so, focus your attention on your thoughts, feelings and physical sensations. What are you thinking? Which emotions can you detect? How does your body feel?

Don't analyse your thoughts and feelings. Don't attempt to change them. Simply experience them. Awareness is all.

In the second part of the meditation, concentrate on your breathing. Follow the steady rise and fall of your chest and diaphragm as you inhale and exhale. If you become distracted, simply guide your mind back to your breathing.

For the third and final minute, broaden your awareness so that you notice how your whole body feels when you breathe. Once again, don't judge these physical sensations – there is no right or wrong way to be feeling. But if you detect any unpleasant sensations, direct your attention to them. Don't try to make these feelings disappear; instead acknowledge and accept their presence in this moment.

Try practising the breathing space meditation twice a day for a week, or whenever you're feeling particularly stressed, worried or sad.

The relaxation exercises in this chapter are tried and tested. In fact, people have been meditating for thousands of years. Make the exercises a regular feature of your week and scientific studies suggest you too will feel more tranquil, confident and content. Indeed, recent neurological research has shown that mindfulness actually produces positive changes in the brain.

In the following chapter, we turn our attention to what is arguably the single most important influence on our happiness: the quality of our relationships.

CHAPTER 8

Improving your relationships

Over the last fifteen years or so psychologists have carried out a huge amount of research into happiness. From this work, one finding in particular stands out: the stronger our relationships, the happier we're likely to be.

That's not to say well-being requires dozens of friends and a frenetic social life. Nor is it dependent on being married or in a long-term relationship, though that can certainly help. When it comes to relationships, quality is far more important than quantity. Research shows that simply having a best friend you can talk to openly and rely upon to help when needed is enough to make all the difference. Having a couple of other close friends will make you happier still.

Of course we all differ in terms of how many relationships we need to be happiest and of what type. But whether we're tremendously outgoing or relatively self-contained, we all need to be loved and supported and to love and support others in turn.

Psychologists have found that the most important benefits of close relationships – romantic or otherwise – include:

- Companionship: having someone to spend time with.
- Self-validation: having someone who is encouraging, supportive and complimentary.
- Help: both practical assistance and general guidance.
- Intimacy: being able to share your most personal thoughts and feelings.
- Trust and loyalty: being able to rely on your friend.
- Emotional security: having someone who's there for you in new and scary situations.

So don't become too isolated. When people are feeling down or very stressed they often turn inwards. Social contact can seem unappealing when you're lacking confidence or energy. You might not be able to face sharing your thoughts with those closest to you. But keeping the lines of communication open, and spending time with the people you like and love, will do wonders for your mood. This chapter will show you how to make the most of your relationships.

> " *spending time with the people you like and love, will do wonders for your mood.* "

Of course, if there are people in your life who make you unhappy in whatever way, you may want to reduce your level of contact. If they're important to you, it's best to bite the bullet and explain how you feel. Very possibly, they're unaware of the effect they're having on you. Explaining your feelings gives them the opportunity to change their behaviour. But whether you opt for the heart-to-heart or simply steer clear of someone, don't feel guilty. You have a right to choose the company of the people who make you feel better and not worse.

In the second part of this chapter we focus on romantic relationships, but let's start with a look at how to develop better relationships with family, friends and colleagues.

BUILDING YOUR SOCIAL NETWORK

What sweetness remains in life if you take away friendship? Depriving life of friendship is like depriving the world of the sun. Friendship is the only thing in the world whose usefulness all humankind are agreed upon. MARCUS TULLIUS CICERO, 384–322 BC

You may remember that in Chapter 4 we suggested you keep an activities diary for a week. It's a record of what you're doing and how you're feeling.

Have a look back at your diary now. How much time did you spend in the company of friends and family? If you haven't had a chance yet to compile an activities diary, start now (see p. 49 for details of how to do it).

Your task for the coming week is simple: spend more time with the people who make you happy! Don't wait for it to happen: go ahead and arrange a meeting or plan an activity to do together. Over the coming weeks, make a note of how much time you're devoting to social activities. Try to build it up gradually and ask yourself whether you notice a change in your mood.

As well as working to develop your existing relationships, if you often find you have no one to spend time with, aim to add to your circle of friends. Who do you know that you'd like to become friends with? Get to know that person better by chatting to them when you can. Suggest that you meet up some time – perhaps you could have a coffee together or see a movie. Take a deep breath and suspend your fears of rejection. More often than not, they're going to be delighted and flattered. Wouldn't you be? It's a natural human instinct to warm to the people who are pleasant to us, so your friendliness is very likely to be reciprocated. And boy will you feel good when it is.

If you're struggling to meet people, consider joining a class or club. Whatever your interest, you can be pretty sure there's a group meeting nearby. Whether it's learning a language, reading books, gardening, yoga, cooking or participating in sports, people love combining their chosen activity with social contact.

Not only is it fun to pursue an interest or hobby as part of a group – which will boost your happiness levels in itself – you instantly have something in common with the other people attending. Those first chats with people we don't know can seem tricky, but this way you'll have a readymade topic for conversation.

Attending for the first time can be daunting, but remember that it's perfectly normal to feel apprehensive when meeting new people. That nervousness will soon pass, and probably within a very few minutes of arriving.

If you're finding it difficult to take the plunge, try to put your finger on what it is that's holding you back. Then focus on the benefits – the reasons why you want to join the group. Write them down so you can remind yourself if you're wavering. And when you do attend, treat yourself to something nice as a reward for your courage.

THE RULES OF FRIENDSHIP

Each friend represents a world in us, a world possibly not born until they arrive, and it is only by this meeting that a new world is born. ANAIS NIN

There's now clear evidence from a number of research studies that friendships – and particularly having a best friend – can make a big difference to our level of happiness, no matter whether we're naturally gregarious or relatively shy, generally content or often unhappy. As we've seen, there are many reasons why having friends makes us feel happier, but some experts believe companionship and self-validation are most important for happiness.

And yet, although friendship is so important to us, it can be a bit of a puzzle. After all, were you taught how to make friends? Did anyone ever sit you down and explain what makes a friendship thrive? For most people, friendship is something we're left to figure out for ourselves – and often we have to learn the hard way.

But the more we understand how friendships work, the better equipped we are to ensure our own relationships are successful. So take a look now at the 'Rules of Friendship'; they came about when the British psychologists Michael Argyle and

Monika Henderson asked people in the UK, Italy, Hong Kong and Japan to define the ingredients of a flourishing friendship:

> *the more we understand how friendships work, the better equipped we are to ensure our own relationships are successful.*

- Volunteer help in time of need.
- Respect the other's privacy.
- Keep confidences.
- Trust and confide in each other.
- Stand up for the other person in their absence.
- Don't criticise each other in public.
- Show emotional support.
- Look him/her in the eye during conversation.
- Strive to make him/her happy while in each other's company.
- Don't be jealous or critical of each other's relationships.
- Be tolerant of each other's friends.
- Share news of success with the other.
- Ask for personal advice.
- Don't nag.
- Engage in joking or teasing with the friend.
- Seek to repay debts and favours and compliments.
- Disclose personal feelings or problems to the friend.

Spend a little time reflecting on your own friendships. Which aspects are you strong at, and which do you think you could do better?

FIVE TECHNIQUES TO STRENGTHEN YOUR RELATIONSHIPS

Some people go to priests; others to poetry; I to my friends. VIRGINIA WOOLF

Building on the rules of friendship, here are five key techniques for a better relationship. Select one as a priority, and find ways to implement it in your friendships. When you feel the time is right, try another technique.

Incidentally, we've included this section in the part of the chapter that focuses on non-romantic relationships, but all five techniques are relevant to romantic relationships too.

Express your gratitude

We've already looked at why and how being grateful is good for you (pp. 72–4), but it's also vital for developing the strongest, most beneficial relationships. There are two forms of gratitude that need attention – we could call them internal and external gratitude. Imagine, for instance, that a friend phones to ask whether you're free to meet up for dinner at the weekend. You have a great time and the next day send them a card, email or text message to say how happy you are to have been asked, and how much you've enjoyed the evening. Simple manners, for sure, but easy to forget in the rush of daily life.

As well as this external form of gratitude, don't neglect the internal. Let yourself enjoy the memory of the evening. Remind yourself how grateful you are to have such a good friend, and to have had the opportunity to share a meal in their company. If you're currently keeping a gratitude journal, note down your feelings there.

Your friendship will be strengthened by both the external and internal forms of gratitude. Everyone likes being thanked (as long as the gratitude is genuine), so your friend is certain to feel even more positively about you. And by reflecting on your gratitude, you'll remind yourself of the value you place on that friendship, and the importance of maintaining it.

Make praise a habit

When was the last time you praised a friend?

If you're struggling to think of an example, don't worry. For many of us, giving praise – just like communicating heartfelt gratitude – doesn't come naturally. This is a pity, because reciprocal praise and admiration can play a huge role in helping relationships to flourish. (The praise has to be real, of course; fake it and you'll be fooling no one.)

We can all learn to make praise a habit. For the next seven days aim to praise at least one person each day. Who it is doesn't matter: it could be your partner, a friend, a family member or colleague. How do the people you praise react? Do you notice a difference in your own mood?

Remember what makes your friend special

When you've known someone a while, it's easy to take them for granted. To breathe new life into a friendship, take the time to remind yourself why you were drawn to this person in the first place.

Jot down on a piece of paper three of your friend's positive qualities (feel free to write more if you'd like). It could be a personality trait such as kindness or optimism, or a talent like playing a musical instrument or cooking wonderfully. Then for each positive quality add an example – a brief note of a time when your friend demonstrated this characteristic.

Notice how your feelings for your friend are revived, and how much you appreciate their unique talents and attributes. Doesn't your friendship seem suddenly much more precious than it did just a few minutes ago? And, building on our suggestions about the importance of gratitude and praise, why not let your friend know how you feel?

Be helpful

In Chapter 4 we introduced the '5 a day' activities for happiness. As part of this programme we recommended giving time to others – in other words, helping the people around us.

When you read those pages, you may have been surprised to learn that helping others is a remarkably effective means of boosting your own well-being. But you'll not be amazed to hear that it's also a great way of building friendships. So ask yourself what you can do to help someone you know – and then go ahead and do it!

Respond positively to good news

> *Anybody can sympathise with the sufferings of a friend, but it requires a very fine nature to sympathise with a friend's success.* OSCAR WILDE

Imagine that you are having coffee with a friend. With a huge smile, she announces that she and her husband are spending the weekend in Paris. How should you react?

The strongest relationships are built on what's called an 'active and constructive' response to good news. That means listening attentively, maintaining eye contact and generally being as positive about the news as your friend is.

By reacting like this, rather than seeming uninterested or unenthusiastic, you demonstrate how much you value your friend's happiness. You show that their pleasure gives you pleasure, thereby reinforcing the bond between you.

How do you typically respond to other people's good news? If it isn't always in an active and constructive manner, make a point of reacting like that in future. It doesn't have to be only the big stuff: whether your friend has become engaged or is simply pleased with a new haircut, whether they've been promoted at work or just had a fun time at the weekend, try to respond with genuine pleasure and enthusiasm. Let your 'very fine nature' shine through!

ROMANTIC RELATIONSHIPS

> *Of all the gods Love is the best friend of humankind, the helper and the healer of all ills that stand in the way of human happiness.* PLATO

When researchers ask people what makes them happy, romantic relationships tend to figure prominently. The psychological research bears this out: a flourishing relationship really can do wonders for the overall happiness of the individuals involved (just as a struggling relationship can undermine it).

> *a flourishing relationship really can do wonders for the overall happiness of the individuals involved*

Romantic relationships can bring many benefits, from intimacy to practical help, sexual fulfillment to enhanced self-esteem. But interestingly, research has suggested that there are two aspects in particular that make for happiness. These are *companionship* – that's to say, having someone to be with – and *emotional security*, or having someone to turn to in difficult times.

The laws of attraction

It's not very romantic to point it out, but falling in love (or making friends) isn't always as mysterious a process as it might seem. In fact, psychologists have discovered that attraction is usually the result of just four key factors.

By becoming aware of these factors, you're in a great position to judge which people you're most likely to be compatible with. And that's going to increase your chances of starting – and maintaining – a successful relationship.

Proximity:

The single most important factor in determining who we get to know, like and even love is simply how much we see of them.

Why does proximity exert such a powerful influence on our feelings? Well, if you run into someone regularly, they soon become pretty familiar. And most of us prefer the familiar to the unfamiliar.

Seeing a lot of someone, of course, also gives us a chance to discover what we like about them, and to build a relationship. And if we know we're likely to be in regular contact, we're more likely to make an effort to get along.

Similarity:

There are exceptions, of course, but most people gravitate towards those who are like them – in intelligence, social class, personality, beliefs, racial background, looks and even weight. We also tend to like people who are of a similar age, though when it comes to long-term partners both sexes prefer the man to be a little older than the woman.

Physical attractiveness:

Men tend to prefer women who are younger than themselves, who wear their hair long, and who are neither very overweight nor especially thin. When it comes to a woman's figure, men go for curves. Women, on the other hand, generally like their men to possess a narrow waist and relatively broad shoulders. Women and men both agree that the male partner should be taller than the female.

When it comes to faces, men and women alike seek out symmetry, proportionality and 'normal' features. That's to say, we tend to prefer the average face to the unusual one.

Of course, these are broad generalisations. As we all know, people vary enormously in the kind of looks they find appealing. And while appearance undoubtedly plays a part in attraction, other influences are arguably far more significant. For instance, research shows that what both men and women value above all in a long-term partner isn't beauty but rather intelligence, kindness, empathy, dependability and love.

Reciprocity:

Simply put, we like those who like us. And because we tend to get back what we give, acting positively towards someone encourages more of the same in return. Behave as though someone likes you and there's a good chance they soon will.

The power of reciprocity was demonstrated in a classic experiment carried out in the mid-1980s. When individuals were led to believe (falsely) that the people they were chatting to liked them a lot, they responded accordingly, displaying much more warmth, openness and all-round friendliness than if they were told (equally falsely) that their companions didn't care for them.

HOW TO STRENGTHEN YOUR ROMANTIC RELATIONSHIP

Tis sweet to know there is an eye will mark our coming, and look brighter when we come. LORD BYRON, *DON JUAN*

Love can sometimes seem like the little girl in the nursery rhyme – when it's good it's very, very good, but when it's bad it's horrid.

We shouldn't be surprised by the occasional rough patch. Maintaining a successful long-term relationship is a complex business that requires lots of time and effort. According to Robin Dunbar, a professor of evolutionary anthropology at Oxford University, this is why it's the birds and mammals that are monogamous that have the biggest brains. So don't worry if your relationship has its ups and downs: it's normal. That said, there's much you can do to ensure the ups far outnumber the downs.

Research suggests that the strongest romantic relationships are based on:

- Shared decision-making
- Trust
- Intimacy – physical, emotional and psychological
- Sexual attraction
- Time and energy working at the relationship
- Agreement about who does which household chores
- Emotional support for each other
- Positive actions, whether it be giving your partner a hug, bringing them a cup of tea in bed, or being ready to listen when they need to talk
- Clear communication
- Tolerance, flexibility and patience
- Negotiation skills

How does your relationship match up to this ideal? Are there particular aspects that you think you should work at?

> Love doesn't sit there like a stone, it has to be made, like bread; remade all of the time, made new. URSULA K. LE GUIN

If you're unhappy with the way your relationship is going right now, try the suggestions below. But also have a look back at the 'Rules of friendship' and 'Five techniques to improve your relationships' sections in the first part of this chapter. They are as relevant to romantic partnerships as they are to any other kind of relationship.

Make time for fun together.
Many relationships suffer because of simple neglect. When partners don't spend enough quality time together, it's easy for them to become remote from one another.

So think back to the things you used to enjoy as a couple – going out to the cinema, staying in bed till noon, buying each other little gifts – and do them again, or schedule in other activities you both think you might enjoy. Plan ahead and make a date, just as you did when you first got together.

Lead by example.

Changing someone else's behaviour can be difficult (though the strategies we present here will certainly help). It's much easier to focus on your own actions.

> *Changing someone else's behaviour can be difficult; it's much easier to focus on your own actions.*

Have a think about your attitudes to the relationship and to handling conflict. Where did they come from? Are you perhaps merely following the example your parents gave you? Could you do things differently? If you can change your own behaviour for the better, you'll probably find your partner will make a similar adjustment.

Don't mind-read.

Many of the conflicts in relationships occur because one partner assumes they know what the other is thinking. And it can be a vicious circle. Mind-reading causes arguments, which in turn can poison the atmosphere between partners and prompt them to think the worst of each other, leading to even more disputes. When a relationship is going through a sticky patch, misunderstandings tend to be rife.

So don't jump to conclusions. If your partner is behaving in a way that troubles you, think through all the possible explanations. *Don't take things personally* – your partner's emotions or actions probably have nothing at all to do with you. When you're calm, let your partner know how you interpreted their behaviour and find out from them what was really going on.

Talk through your mutual expectations.

We all bring a lot of baggage to a relationship. We have strong views about everything from how the household should run to what kind of sex life we expect. Lots of this baggage comes from our upbringing and previous relationships. Some of it may stem from our gender: men and women often have very different approaches to the various issues that crop up in a relationship (not least of which is how to handle arguments).

So it's really important to have an honest discussion with your partner about your expectations for the relationship. Who's going to clean the house? Who is responsible for childcare? How will you handle the finances? How much 'personal' time should you each have? What are your respective views on fidelity, commitment and trust?

Remember that it's not a question of winning an argument. The aim is to understand and respect where you're each coming from, and to reach an agreement on how you'll proceed in the future. If you're lucky, you'll agree on most things; more likely, you'll both need to compromise.

Work at your communication skills.

It's pretty much impossible for a relationship to thrive if the communication within it is poor. So if you take nothing else away from these pages, remember these guidelines:

- *Talk to one another!* Let your partner know how you're feeling, discuss how you think the relationship is going, whether your needs and expectations have changed, and work together to solve problems (for more on problem-solving techniques, see p. 59).

- *Be clear and specific* about what's troubling you. Resist the temptation to make sweeping, general complaints ('You never lift a finger around the house'). Instead, focus on the particular ('We need to work out a rota for the washing up and the vacuuming').

- *Let your partner talk.* No matter how badly you want to get things off your chest, don't rant on. Be as calm and measured as you can, and keep it short and sweet and to the point. Leave gaps for your partner to speak.

- *Be positive.* No one likes being criticised, so don't focus on the negative aspects of your partner's behaviour. Instead, present your requests in terms of positive actions you'd like them to take. For example, instead of 'You're always undermining me', try 'I'd like you to back me up even if you don't always agree.'

  Remember that the best way of changing someone's behaviour isn't to criticise what you don't like; it's to praise and encourage what you do like.

- *Use 'I' and 'we', not 'you'.* Don't point the finger at your partner ('You're always...', 'You never...'); be up front about your own wishes ('I'd like...', 'I think we need to...'). It's a way of signalling that you're willing to take your share of the responsibility for solving the problem, rather than simply blaming your partner. Using 'we' will work wonders too: a subtle but eloquent sign that you want to work together to sort things out.

- *Remember that communication is not simply about the things you say.* It's the hugs and kisses, the smiles and caresses and the willingness to make eye contact – in other words, the full range of non-verbal signals that we're constantly sending out to our partner.

- *Show your partner that you're really listening to what they have to say* by your facial expression, the nod of your head, the words you use and the actions you take. Simply recapping what your partner has told you will help enormously ('I understand that you're exhausted after your day at work and that you don't want to cook every night.').

  Equally important is that you work at *empathising* with your partner. This means trying to think yourself into their position and share their feelings.

- *Call a truce.* When things are really difficult, it can help to call a truce. Both partners agree to discuss their differences at a set time, in a comfortable, quiet and private place, without being rude or aggressive or hostile. One partner talks for five minutes while the other listens carefully and respectfully. Then the other partner has their turn.

  Generally ten minutes is enough to begin with, though you may want to build up to twenty minutes. Hold these discussions regularly, but don't discuss your problems in the meantime. Putting your thoughts in a letter is another technique that people have found useful.

- *Listen!* This is arguably the most important communication skill of all. Give your partner the space and time to tell you what's on their mind. Don't interrupt; don't mind-read; and don't let your attention wander. Try not to dismiss what they say; be open-minded and flexible. Make listening your priority.

Negotiate!

Winning an argument with your partner may feel like a victory, but in fact all you're probably doing is breeding frustration, anger and resentment. So aim to end your arguments with agreement and compromise. The best way to achieve that is by polishing up your negotiation skills:

- *Don't complain: request.* Moaning may feel good, but it won't bring the kind of change you're looking for. Try specific – and realistic – requests instead. For example, rather than complaining that your partner doesn't help out with the childcare, ask that he bath the kids three times a week. It's better to set modest targets that can be met than wildly optimistic ones that can only end in failure.

- *Be clear about what you want.* It can be difficult to say what's really on our mind, but if we don't problems are likely to continue. Don't make it a test of your partner's sensitivity: help them out by explaining calmly and clearly how you feel.

- *Focus on the future, not on the past.* Raking over past issues isn't going to create the sense of positive, cooperative problem-solving that strong relationships need. So let go of what you can't change and concentrate on what you can: the future.

- *Give and take.* If you're asking your partner to do something they might rather avoid (washing the car, tidying the house, visiting your family), it'll help if you can offer something positive in return. This is negotiation: finding a solution that balances each partner's needs and desires. Or, in other words, give and take.

- *Timetable.* This can be a great way of ensuring everyone's requirements are met. For example, if you're concerned that your partner spends all their free time on the Internet instead of with you, schedule a night out together every week and, in return, agree that your partner can surf the web for a couple of hours two evenings a week.

If all this feels too formal and unspontaneous, remember that there's no need to timetable your every waking moment, just the activities that matter to you both. And once you've both got used to the new way of doing things, you probably won't need the timetable.

Defuse arguments before they get out of hand.

If tempers begin to flare, there's still lots you can do to stop things developing into a full-blown row:

> *Speak when you are angry and you will make the best speech you will ever regret.* AMBROSE BIERCE

- Don't be hostile or aggressive, and stay clear of sarcasm. The 'sting in the tail' – a negative comment at the end of a positive message – can be particularly damaging.

- Be sensitive to the fact that the argument is escalating. Learn to recognise the signs, perhaps in the way that you're feeling or how you and your partner are interacting. Step outside the conflict and ask your partner whether he's noticed what's happening.

- Speak more quietly and slowly.

- Relax. Count to ten, or practise deep breathing.

- Reach out to your partner. Shift the mood by smiling, or giving your partner a hug. Humour can be effective – as long as you're sure your partner will find your comment funny.

- Be prepared to apologise (provided you really mean it).

● If things are getting really heated, call a time out. Separate for at least twenty minutes and then come back together to discuss things calmly.

Be clear about whether you want to remain in the relationship.
If things are really difficult between you and your partner, you may need to decide whether it's worth staying together. But before you do anything drastic, consider seeing a relationship counsellor. The Relate organisation runs a nationwide network of counsellors, though your GP may also be able to recommend a suitable person. And talk things over with trusted friends. Weigh up the pros and cons, both of remaining in the relationship and splitting up. Don't base your decision on how you feel right now; imagine how things might be in three, six, or twelve months' time.

A brief word about sex

A lively sex life isn't an essential part of a successful relationship, especially for couples that have been together for a while. On the other hand, sex can provide pleasure, excitement and intimacy, and an opportunity for each partner to reaffirm their love and desire for one another.

Whatever the place of sex in your relationship – central, marginal or somewhere in between – all is fine as long as both you and your partner are content with the status quo. If that changes, though, you have an issue that needs to be tackled.

Of course many of us find sex an awkward topic to discuss at the best of times. And it doesn't get any easier when things aren't going well. But this is definitely a nettle that must be grasped. Let your partner know what's on your mind. Only then will you be able to work together to find a solution.

On pp. 143–4 you'll find brief notes on the most common sexual problems. Several excellent books are available to help tackle these problems; you'll find them listed, together with our advice on overcoming these difficulties, in our book *Know Your*

Mind (see Further Reading, p. 157). Very probably that'll be all you need to get your sex life back on track. But if things don't improve, contact a sex therapist or relationship counsellor. Your GP should be able to provide a recommendation.

Human beings are intensely social creatures. Whatever our personality – whether we're extremely gregarious or generally happy with our own company – our emotional life revolves around the people we know, like and love.

It stands to reason then that improving those relationships can provide a massive boost to our well-being. Introduce the exercises and activities in this chapter to your routine and you'll discover just how big a difference they can make.

CHAPTER 9

Happiness at work

For most of us, work is a fundamental part of life. When it's good it can provide us with everything from fulfilment to friends. But when things aren't working out, it's something best not ignored.

Work occupies such a large proportion of our time that it's hardly surprising how much of a powerful influence it exerts on our level of happiness. It's possible, of course, to be happy at work and unhappy in other aspects of life – and vice versa. But the scientific data suggests that people who are happy at work are happier all round.

When you think about it, this isn't surprising. Positive emotions have a nice habit of spilling over from one part of our life to another. If we find our work enjoyable, rewarding and satisfying, those feelings of contentment are likely to stay with us even when we're not in the office.

Hold on, you might be thinking at this point: that's a very big 'if'. But you don't have to possess your dream job to find happiness at work. Granted, if you're really miserable at work it may well be time to explore other options (see p. 130), but if things haven't reached that stage, there's a lot you can do to increase your level of fun, interest and fulfilment.

WHAT MAKES PEOPLE HAPPY AT WORK?

Before we get stuck into what you can *do* to boost your work feelgood factor, it's worth having a look at what the evidence suggests contributes most to job satisfaction.

The following list was compiled by Peter Warr, a psychologist who specialises in employment issues. It's the product of many years of research and countless surveys.

As you read it through, reflect on your own experiences at work. Which of the factors are most important to you? Which are you missing right now? And can you think of ideas to rectify the shortfall?

- **Influence:** Possessing at least some control over your work.

- **Skills:** Being able to utilise your existing skills and having the chance to develop new ones.

- **Demands:** Having challenging, but achievable, goals.

- **Variety:** Not being expected to perform the same task, in the same place and in the same way, every day.

- **Requirements:** Understanding what's needed from you and how to go about delivering it.

- **Positive relationships:** Enjoying sufficient social contact (as with all these factors, exactly how much is enough will vary from person to person), and friendly, supportive, enjoyable relationships.

- **Money:** Being well rewarded for your efforts.

- **Environment:** A safe and comfortable workplace.

- **Meaning:** A role you believe is valuable and that is respected both by colleagues and society at large.

- **Management:** A boss you can rely upon for advice and support.

- **Career:** Being confident that your job is secure, and that you can progress to a different role when you're ready.

- **Fairness:** Believing that the people you work for are honourable, honest and trustworthy.

THE BENEFITS OF HAPPINESS AT WORK

Feeling happier in your job brings an immediate and very obvious reward. You feel much better! But as if that weren't sufficient, research indicates that people who are happy at work:

> *Feeling happier in your job brings an immediate and very obvious reward. You feel much better!*

- Perform more effectively
- Are more motivated, energetic and enthusiastic
- Get on better with colleagues and customers
- Earn higher salaries
- Receive more promotions and bonuses
- Take less time off sick
- Stay with the organisation for longer

None of these is likely to be your main motivation as you set about increasing your happiness at work. But they're a very pleasant fringe benefit. And when you've thought about the kind of changes that would improve your situation at work, they may also help secure your boss's buy-in. After all, if you explain to your manager that the changes would make you more motivated and enthusiastic, and would help improve your productivity and performance, they're more likely to sit up and take notice.

How to become happier at work

Far and away the best prize that life offers is the chance to work hard at work worth doing. THEODORE ROOSEVELT

Strengthen your relationships

As you'll know from reading Chapter 8, nothing is more important for happiness than our relationships. That goes for work too. You may spend more time with your colleagues than you do with your friends, family, or even partner. So getting along well can make a huge difference to how you feel about work in general.

Compare and contrast how you'd feel in these two real-life workplaces.

In office A, most members of staff have their own small office. This might be regarded as a perk, but in reality it's more of a curse. Individuals rarely emerge from their offices and consequently hardly know many of their colleagues. Moreover, since it's a sandwich-at-the-desk culture, even lunch rarely provides an opportunity for social contact. Visits to the pub after work are almost unheard of. The hours can drag.

Now imagine doing the same job in a very different company. This time the office is open plan, the atmosphere open and gregarious. Lunch is eaten together, either in the company canteen or occasionally at a local pub. Social activities are regularly arranged for evenings – meals out, trips to concerts or comedy clubs, annual summer and Christmas parties. Colleagues develop into friends. Work becomes fun.

The second job is likely to be many, many times more enjoyable than the first, even though the day-to-day details of the role are more or less identical. When work is a place where we get to hang out with friends, it can suddenly seem like rather a nice way to spend the day.

But what if we find ourselves working with people with whom we don't hit it off, or in an organisation that doesn't place a priority on sociability? Well, as Mahatma Gandhi explained: 'You must be the change you wish to see in the world.' That means striving to display the kind of behaviour and attitude you hope for from your colleagues.

The psychologist Christopher Chris Peterson argues that positive team spirit is fostered by the following behaviours:

- Showing commitment to whichever task you're engaged in.

- Resisting the temptation to moan or show frustration.

- Pulling your weight – and more.

- Volunteering to take on responsibility.

- Praising your team-mates.

- Helping other team members and the team leader achieve their goals.

More generally, ask yourself what you can do to make your workplace a more enjoyable place to be. If you're friendly, open and helpful, there's a very good chance that the people around you will begin to behave in that way too. Don't neglect your communication skills (see p. 111). And if at first it doesn't seem to be working, keep going. Sooner or later the ice will thaw!

For advice on how to go about building relationships, have a look back at Chapter 8.

COMMIT TO YOUR JOB

There is nothing so satisfying to the spirit, so defining of our character than giving our all to a difficult task.
BARACK OBAMA

Can you recall a time when you were overworked in your job, rushed off your feet for days on end? At the other end of the spectrum, have you ever found yourself with too little to do, struggling to fill the hours until you can finally head home? Which of the two situations did you find most stressful?

Clearly, having too much to do is no fun, at least over the long term. But research suggests that for most people it's preferable to the opposite scenario. As employment guru Jessica Pryce-Jones puts it: 'Hard work leads to happiness.' We're most content in our jobs – and indeed in other areas of our life – when we're getting things done.

Frequently, of course, it's not a lack of tasks that reduces our productivity but our attitude towards those tasks. Everyone experiences occasional days when they're just not in the mood for work. But if you're feeling like that on a regular basis, it's time to do something about it.

Step one is a psychological shift. Recalling the great Bill Shankly, his former manager at Liverpool, the footballer Kevin Keegan commented: 'I learned so much from Shanks. He used to say: "If I was a road-sweeper, my street would be the cleanest in the borough." I took that to heart.' So don't fight work; give yourself up to it. Resolve to perform every task, no matter how trivial, to the best of your ability. The old adage is true: the more you put in, the more you'll get out.

> *If a man is called a streetsweeper, he should sweep streets
> even as Michelangelo painted, or Beethoven composed music,
> or Shakespeare wrote poetry. He should sweep streets so
> well that all the hosts of heaven and Earth will pause to say,
> Here lived a great streetsweeper who did his job well.*
> MARTIN LUTHER KING, JR.

Step two is a practical technique. If you can increase your productivity you'll feel so much better about yourself and your job. Achievement feels wonderful. And the best way to boost your productivity is to set yourself realistic goals: for example, by the end of next week I will have dealt with x or done the research for y or investigated z. By November I will have put forward my proposal for re-organising the computing systems or changing how we handle complaints or .... You get the idea. The best goals are:

- **Challenging but feasible.** The most highly motivated people set themselves relatively tricky (though still attainable) goals; they thrive when required to raise their game.

- **Clear, specific and measurable.** You need to understand exactly what's required, how to achieve it and how you'll know when it's been completed.

- **Attainable quickly.** Any goal that requires many weeks or months to achieve is likely to require superhuman levels of motivation. It's easy to feel discouraged if that end point still seems ages away after lots of effort. So if your goal requires sustained input, identify lots of smaller subgoals that will help you reach your overall objective – and give yourself a little reward as you achieve them.

Goals aren't just a great way to help you get more done. You'll find that simply defining your goals and tracking your progress gives you a sense of control – which, as we've just seen, is one of the key factors in determining job satisfaction (you'll find more on boosting your level of control at work on p. 126). Just thinking up goals can be enormously empowering. Making progress with them will bring even more positive feelings.

> *simply defining your goals and tracking your progress gives you a sense of control*

FIND MEANING IN YOUR WORK

Steve Jobs was co-founder of Apple Inc, the largest technology company in the world, which he helped set up at the age of twenty-one. Here is Steve Jobs' career advice:

You've got to find what you love and that is as true for work as it is for lovers. Your work is going to fill a large part of your life and the only way to be truly satisfied is to do what you believe is great work. And the only way to do great work is to love what you do. If you haven't found it yet, keep looking and don't settle. As with all matters of the heart, you'll know when you've found it.

Jobs may have been overstating the case a bit, but there's no doubt that if you love your work, if you believe it is worth doing, you'll be happy in your role. That doesn't mean, of course, that you won't sometimes experience setbacks. But when you do you'll know why it's important to keep going regardless. And you'll be better able to overcome those challenges.

Research has shown that people tend to view their work in one of three ways. A *job* is a chore we endure simply for the money. A *career* is work that we may or may not enjoy, but for which our primary motivation is advancement – for example, money, recognition and status. A *calling*, on the other hand, is a role we find rewarding in itself. A calling is what Steve Jobs was describing in the quote above. Katharine Graham, long-time publisher of the *Washington Post*, put it more succinctly: 'To love what you do and feel that it matters – how could anything be more fun?'

The trick, then, is to turn your job into a calling. But is this really possible if we're clinging onto whatever employment we can find in a fraught economic climate; if we've never found the work that is our passion; or if we know what we'd really love to be doing, but find ourselves stuck with something quite different?

Well, some roles, of course, suit us better than others. Some jobs we find relatively easy to love. But even for those of us not doing our dream job, there are steps we can take to make our role less like a job and more like a calling.

The first is to build on your strengths, values and skills. As we saw in Chapter 4, *strengths* are positive character traits and behaviours, such as creativity, teamwork, self-discipline, leadership, persistence and kindness. *Values* are what we believe is important in life. (See pp. 44–6 for more on strengths and values.) *Skills*, on the other hand, are techniques you learn and master through practice – for example, giving a successful presentation, writing a persuasive email, or dealing positively with a customer.

Take the time to understand your strengths, values and skills (you'll find a questionnaire on strengths at www. viasurvey.org). If possible, choose a job that fits well with them. And if you're already in a job, see what you can do to reshape your role accordingly. If you're creative, for instance, is there any task you could take on that would allow you to use this strength? If you're good with people, how could you increase this element of your work? If you value equality and justice, strive to promote these values in your dealings with your colleagues or customers.

> *Your work is to discover your work and then, with all your heart, to give yourself to it.* BUDDHA

Crafting your role to suit you better may require the support of your manager. But you don't need anyone else's buy-in to reshape your *attitude* to work. With a change of perspective, you can find new meaning in your role, whatever it happens to be.

> **With a change of perspective, you can find new meaning in your role, whatever it happens to be.**

Committing to your job, as we described above, is a great start. To help you, think of five positive reasons for doing what you do.

Kirsty is a 34-year-old PA to a company director. It's a role she fell into, largely because she couldn't think of anything else to do. Having experienced periods of disliking her job, Kirsty expected it would be difficult to find five positives. However, here's what she came up with:

- I'm able to provide for my son and daughter.
- I'm good at what I do.
- I enjoy the social contact.
- I'm lucky to have any job at all in the current economic downturn.
- I can fit my job around my other responsibilities and interests.

Write down your positives and keep them handy – maybe pin them up in the kitchen or carry them around with you on a card. If you're feeling negative about work, you'll be able to remind yourself what you're in it for.

And don't forget the techniques in Chapters 5 and 6 for reducing the impact of negative thoughts and increasing positive thoughts. They're just as relevant to the world of work as they are to any other area of life.

The best way to appreciate your job is to imagine yourself without one. OSCAR WILDE

INCREASE YOUR LEVEL OF CONTROL

Research has shown that there's a very clear correlation between the amount of control a person has over their work and their happiness in that role. Broadly speaking, the more control you have, the happier you'll be. That said, everyone has an upper limit. Some people would run the whole show if they could, while others are content simply to manage their own workload. What level of influence are you comfortable with? What level do you have now?

If you're not happy with how things stand at the moment, ask yourself what changes you could make. Talk to your manager about taking on more responsibility, or suggest improvements to the way things currently get done. Increase your influence by upping your involvement in decision-making. It's likely that your manager will welcome your contribution: after all, it's a sign that you care about what you do. And as Jessica Pryce-Jones puts it: 'actively seek out what you can do rather than ruminate on what you can't'.

It's much easier to exert control over our work (and other areas of life) if we've learned how to be assertive. Assertiveness means letting the people around us know how we feel and what we want, clearly, calmly and respectfully.

Assertiveness is especially useful when it comes to saying 'no' – something many of us find exceptionally difficult. Here are some techniques to help you with that tiny but ever so tricky word.

- If you're not sure how you feel about a task, or you don't feel able to say no there and then, buy yourself time. When you're asked to do something, say you'll think it over and get back to them. 'I'd like to just review what else has to be done this week – I'll come back to you later today' is a perfectly reasonable response.

- Be sympathetic and constructive. Tell the person you understand their problem and help them think through alternative solutions – that don't involve you!

- Explain why you can't help, but don't let your reasons sound like excuses. Remember: you are entitled to take control of your own workload.

- Sometimes you may want to meet the person halfway: 'I can't do x, but I may be able to help you with y.'

- With your boss, you can explain that 'I can do this today, if that other task can wait until tomorrow: is that okay?'

Learning to be assertive can be hard, at least at first. It takes courage to speak up for yourself – and you should remember that when you do. Make sure you give yourself the praise you deserve.

DEVELOP YOUR SKILLS

Chapter 4 set out the five a day activities for happiness. One of the five, as you may remember, was learning new skills.

Well, learning is as important for happiness at work as it is in life generally. Most of us want to feel that we're moving forward in our job, becoming better at what we do, developing new skills and adding to our range of experiences.

To help you do this:

- Aim to take on increasingly challenging (though not impossible) assignments. Stretch yourself: not only will you learn lots, the sense of achievement will be a huge morale-boost.

- Consider how you'd like your role to develop over the next year or so, and share your thoughts with your manager. What must happen to make that wish a reality? What training do you need? Which tasks could you take on right now?

- Draw up a plan for what you'd like to be doing in the medium to long term. Do as much research as you can; if you can talk to someone currently in that role so much the better. Find out what skills and experience are required and decide how to go about acquiring them. You may be able to develop aspects of your current job, or it may be a case of taking courses, or building work-related experience in your spare time.

LOOK AFTER YOURSELF

A major cultural shift has occurred in France in recent years. Instead of long, relaxing, restaurant lunches, the French worker is now more likely to wolf down a pre-packaged sandwich at their desk. Indeed, the average French lunch break is reported to have shrunk from 90 minutes in 1975 to 32 minutes in 2005.

News of this development was greeted with some amusement in the UK, where it was often seen as a sort of comeuppance for a society finally coming to terms with the real world.

But if there is a lesson to be learned here, it's not that French lunch breaks were too long, but that for most of us they are too short. We'll feel a lot happier at work – and get more done – if we eat a healthy meal and take a decent break from the daily grind.

Working flat out for hours on end is unlikely to increase your well-being, nor will it increase your productivity. All it will do is exhaust you – and no one works well when they're tired. So make sure you take regular breaks during the day. If you can, leave your desk. Even better is to take a brief stroll outside in the fresh air. Enjoy a conversation with a colleague that *isn't* about work.

Meditation can be a fantastic way to relax, even in the most stressful situations. So why not make the three-minute breathing space meditation (see p. 95) a regular part of your working day?

Remember the mini-activities for happiness we discussed on p. 54? Adding five positive activities to your day – no matter how small – will make a real difference to your mood.

Don't let work dominate your life, no matter how rewarding you find it. As the Dalai Lama has written: 'a happy life should have variety … One should not concentrate on job or money'. If we're not careful, work can swallow up the time we should be spending with friends and family, or on hobbies and pastimes, or even sleeping. So make these your priority; work will take care of itself.

If at all possible, try to keep your working day within sensible limits. Bar a very few jobs, by law no one in the UK can be forced to work more than 48 hours a week. The average is around 35 hours, which is a much more sensible figure. Of course, there are probably times when the volume of work means that you have to work longer than you'd like. Or perhaps you work in an organisation where long hours are the norm. If you're happy with the situation, that's fine; but if not, it's best to tackle the issue rather than letting it get you down. Start by having a chat with your manager. If that doesn't bear fruit, it may be time to consider making a move.

When things are going badly at work, talking about the situation with family or friends is often the last thing we want to do. Instead, we try to build a wall between work and the other parts of our life. But of course problems at work don't tend to stay there. Instead, they can dominate our thoughts and drag down our mood, no matter where we are. So don't bottle up your concerns: talk them through with the people closest to you.

If you are too busy to spend time with your children,
then you are busier than God intended you to be.
RABBI MENDEL EPSTEIN

The techniques we've described here should provide a real boost to your level of contentment at work. But if you've given them a good try and are still unhappy, it may be time to consider changing jobs.

If you're in that position, take the time to plan your next move properly. Investigate the possibilities as thoroughly as possible. Talk the issues through with your friends and loved ones; perhaps consult a careers adviser. Which roles would suit your strengths, values and skills? What do you need to add to your portfolio to maximise your chances of landing the right job? Are you confident you'll feel happier in that role than in your current position?

Changing jobs presents a big opportunity to become happier at work. If it takes a while to come to a decision, that's just as it ought to be. The prize is definitely worth the effort.

CHAPTER 10

Underlying problems: common psychological issues that fuel unhappiness

At the beginning of *You Can Be Happy* we introduced the four components of well-being. One of the four doesn't tend to feature in books about happiness, but we believe the evidence suggests it's as important as any of the others. That component is 'fewer negative emotions', and in Chapter 5 we set out some of the techniques you can use to achieve this.

But negative emotions are often fuelled by specific psychological problems, such as worry, stress and feeling down or depressed. In this chapter we look at the most common types of psychological problems. Perhaps you'll recognise a trigger for your own unhappiness in one or other of them, and when you've recognised it, you'll be in a much better position to deal with it.

If your unhappiness does happen to have its roots in one of these common problems, you'll almost certainly find that tackling that problem is enough to bring about a considerable improvement in your well-being.

All of the problems we discuss in this chapter exist on a spectrum. This means that the impact they have on individuals varies hugely. Some people are affected quite severely, while lots more experience relatively mild difficulties. If you're at the mild end now, that *doesn't* mean you're going to end up at the severe end later. Often things get better simply with the passage of time, but if you're finding life tough there's a lot you can do to speed up the process.

Admitting you may have a problem, and seeking help for it, can be scary. It doesn't help that although psychological problems are incredibly widespread, most people don't like to talk about them. This means that it's easy to feel that you're the only person in the world experiencing difficulties. But as you'll see from the statistics in the following pages, you most definitely are not.

Of course you don't have to tell anyone else what you're going through if you don't want to (though it's often a good idea to make an exception for your doctor). On the other hand, if you do feel able to discuss your feelings with trusted friends and family, you may be surprised to discover that they have much more personal experience of this sort of thing than you think.

Taking the plunge and confronting a problem can be daunting, but you'll be so pleased and proud when you've done so. Not only are these problems extremely common, they are also very treatable. A vast amount of research has been carried out and huge strides made in clinical practice using cognitive behaviour therapy (CBT).

> *Taking the plunge and confronting a problem can be daunting, but you'll be so pleased when you've done so.*

There's no need to put up with things, no need to 'grin and bear it'. For common psychological problems, however much they're troubling you, scientifically proven, highly effective therapies are now available. We discuss how to begin getting help at the end of this chapter.

ANXIETY PROBLEMS

Anxiety can take many forms, here we focus on the six main types:

- Worry
- Phobias
- Panic
- Obsessions and compulsions
- Shyness and social anxiety
- Trauma

Worry

Worry is such a normal part of human experience that the doctor and writer Lewis Thomas once commented: 'We are, perhaps uniquely among the earth's creatures, the worrying animal.'

When we worry, we become preoccupied with an aspect of our life, trying to anticipate what might go wrong and what the consequences will be if it does. People often imagine that worrying helps them deal with issues; unfortunately, it usually has the opposite effect.

That's because worrying and problem-solving are two very different activities. Rather than improving our mood, worrying generally makes us feel worse. Once we start worrying, it can develop into a habit; and if our worrying gets out of hand, life can become very miserable indeed. (The most severe type of worry is called generalised anxiety disorder, or GAD, which affects about 5.7 per cent of people at some point during their lifetime.)

If you're concerned about your worrying, try the Penn State Worry Questionnaire. First, enter the number that describes how typical or characteristic each of the following statements is of you, putting the number next to each one.

1	2	3	4	5
Not at all typical		Somewhat typical		Very typical

1 If I don't have enough time to do everything, I don't worry about it. ____

2 My worries overwhelm me. ____

3 I don't tend to worry about things. ____

4 Many situations make me worry. ____

5 I know I shouldn't worry about things, but I just can't help it. ____

6 When I'm under pressure, I worry a lot. ____

7 I am always worrying about something. ____

8 I find it easy to dismiss worrisome thoughts. ____

9 As soon as I finish one task, I start to worry about something else. ____

10 I never worry about anything. ____

11 When there is nothing more I can do about a concern, I don't worry about it anymore. ____

12 I've been a worrier all my life. ____

13 I notice that I have been worrying about things. ____

14 Once I start worrying, I can't stop. ____

15 I worry all the time. ____

16 I worry about projects until they are all done. __

Source: Meyer, T.J., Miller, M.L., Metzger, R.L. and Borkovec, T.D. 'Development and validation of the Penn State Worry Questionnaire', *Behavioural Research and Therapy*, 28, 487–95, (Elsevier, 1990)

Now add up your scores for each statement. Questions 3, 8, 10, 11 are *reversed scored*: if for example you put 5, for scoring purposes the item is counted as one. Scores can range from 18 to 80.

People with worry problems usually score above 50. A score of over 60 may well indicate GAD, but bear in mind that the questionnaire doesn't provide a diagnosis. Think of it instead as a guide to help you decide whether or not to seek additional help.

Phobias

Aretha Franklin has a fear of flying; Madonna is scared of thunder; and Johnny Depp is reportedly afraid of spiders, ghosts and clowns.

Nearly everyone is afraid of something, and for around 11 per cent of us that fear will at some point develop into a phobia – an intense feeling of fright and anxiety that's out of all proportion to the reality of the threat facing us. Fear of animals, heights, blood, enclosed spaces, water and flying are the most common phobias.

> *Do the thing we fear and death of fear is certain.* RALPH WALDO EMERSON

Panic

For most of us, the word 'panic' describes a sudden feeling of intense anxiety. It's what we experience when we can't find our passport at the airport, or suspect that we've deleted a crucial file on our computer.

Unpleasant though it is, this kind of experience is a very diluted version of the real thing. Genuine panic means being hit by a tsunami of fear, accompanied by a variety of unpleasant physical sensations, such as chest pains, trembling, dizziness and nausea, and terrifying thoughts – for example, that we're about to lose control or faint, that we're going mad, or that we're dying.

Around one in five of us have had an unexpected panic attack, generally when we're very stressed. People who suffer from regular panic attacks may be diagnosed with *panic disorder*. Around 2.7 per cent of the population are estimated to have experienced panic disorder during the past year, with 4.7 per cent of people developing it at some point in their life.

> **Around one in five of us have had an unexpected panic attack**

Obsessions and compulsions

Have you ever left the house and then hurried back, maybe several times, to check you've turned off the cooker? Do you sometimes feel the need to wash your hands repeatedly after going to the toilet or touching something dirty?

How about strange thoughts that pop into your mind as if from nowhere? Do you ever find yourself thinking, for example, that you're about to hit someone? Or shout or swear in the most inappropriate situations – at a church service perhaps, or in a library?

Virtually everyone experiences impulses like this occasionally, but for around 3 per cent of people at some point in their life these normal thoughts and urges spiral out of control: this is *obsessive-compulsive disorder* (OCD).

Shyness and social anxiety

Forty per cent of people describe themselves as shy, and almost everyone has felt shy at some point – especially as children or young adults. Lots of people are perfectly comfortable with their shyness, but it can be pretty severe, and that's no fun at all. When shyness is really pronounced, it's called *social anxiety*.

Social anxiety takes many forms. Some people find all social situations distressing; for others, the fear only kicks in when they have to perform a particular activity in front of others. Most often that activity is public speaking, but social anxiety can concern everything from dating to eating to using a public toilet.

Just like shyness, social anxiety is rooted in the fear that other people will think badly of us. Around 13 per cent of people will experience social anxiety at some stage of their life.

TRAUMA

Psychologists use the term *trauma* to refer to really serious life events, such as rape, violent physical assault, serious illness, natural disasters, a bad car accident, the sudden death of a loved one, a terrorist incident, combat, torture or physical and sexual abuse.

About half of us will experience a severe trauma at some point, and no one takes it in their stride. Being knocked for six is normal and natural. It's the way we deal with a horrible event, working it through in our mind until we get closure and can move on.

In most cases, things begin to improve after a few weeks, but not for everyone; indeed, some people find they're feeling worse than ever. When this happens, it's known as post-traumatic stress disorder (PTSD). Around 5–10 per cent of us are likely to suffer from PTSD at some stage during our lifetime.

DEPRESSION

We all feel down occasionally. Sadness, like happiness, is simply part of life. Generally it lifts pretty quickly, but sometimes the everyday blues take root and deepen into depression.

When people are depressed, life seems devoid of interest or pleasure. They feel exhausted and their concentration span shrinks. Making decisions becomes a nightmare, while completing the most basic task – washing the dishes, phoning a friend, even getting out of bed – seems almost impossible.

Depressed people often lose their appetite, though some resort to comfort feeding. They also frequently have problems sleeping, though again it can work the other way – depression leaves some people listless and sleepy.

Depression changes behaviour, but it also fills the mind with negative thoughts: 'I'm rubbish', 'The world is a bad place', 'I've nothing to look forward to'. People with depression are sometimes wracked by guilt – for past failings and, most especially, for the way they feel now.

Nowadays people are often much more willing to admit to depression, perhaps partly because many celebrities – for example, J.K. Rowling, Alistair Campbell and Stephen Fry – have admitted to battling the illness. Depression is so common that it's been called the 'common cold of the mind'. Around 10–20 per cent of us will experience at least one episode of depression at some point in our lives.

ANGER

Holding anger is like grasping a hot coal with the intent of throwing it at someone else; you are the one who gets burned. BUDDHA

Anger is a perfectly normal and absolutely fundamental emotion. As every parent knows, even the tiniest baby experiences anger – it's part of being human. Whenever we're angry with other people, it always boils down to the same thing: we believe they've done us wrong, or have prevented us from getting what we want, either deliberately or through carelessness.

Although everyone gets annoyed from time to time, it's important that we're able to keep our anger under control. If not, we run the risk of some unpleasant consequences. For example, anger can play havoc with our physical health, making us more susceptible to heart disease and to strokes. It also dramatically increases the chance of us having an accident in the car or at work.

And of course anger and happiness are pretty much incompatible, not least because anger can have such a toxic effect on our relationships. If we're angry much of the time, we're unlikely to be very content. On the other hand, if we can learn to control our anger, happiness is suddenly within reach.

> *anger and happiness are pretty much incompatible: if we're angry much of the time, we're unlikely to be very content.*

STRESS

We all go through periods when life seems a struggle. Perhaps we're trying to balance the demands of our job against the responsibilities of family life. Maybe we're worried about our health or perhaps our relationships are going through a difficult patch, or money is tight.

These are obviously difficult situations, but sometimes we're able to manage pretty well. This is because stress is the result not just of difficult situations, but of our reaction to them: *stress is what we feel when we believe we can't cope with the demands facing us.*

> *stress is what we feel when we believe we can't cope with the demands facing us.*

Typical symptoms of stress include:

- Feeling anxious and tense
- Feeling unable to cope
- Thinking that you've got too much to do

- Feeling under pressure from other people
- Being irritable and grouchy
- Feeling lonely or isolated
- Feeling tired
- Worrying about the future
- Having problems relaxing or sleeping.

Because stress is all about our *response* to potential problems, our ability to cope often depends on how we're feeling at the time. If we're tired or low, we're more likely to think we can't manage and therefore to be much more stressed. A situation that might make us extremely stressed when we're feeling down may hardly affect us when we're well-rested, positive and happy.

Many hundreds of thousands of people in Great Britain suffer from work-related stress every year, with millions of working days lost as a result.

Alcohol problems

Wine is a turncoat; first a friend and then an enemy.
HENRY FIELDING

Human beings have been drinking alcohol for tens of thousands of years – and it's no wonder: for many people, alcohol is a great way to relax, helping us forget our worries and making socialising much easier.

But drinking too much can lead to all manner of physical and psychological problems. In moderation, alcohol can be a source of great pleasure; in excess – and without wanting to sound too preachy – it can cause huge unhappiness.

Judging whether or not you have a problem with alcohol can be hard. Ours is a culture, after all, which regards drinking – even in great quantities – as normal. Many people do drink more than the recommended limits. These are:

- 3–4 units per day for men
- 2–3 units per day for women
- 21 units per week for men
- 14 units per week for women.

It may be time to consider abstaining or cutting down if:

- You regularly drink more than the recommended limits
- You find it difficult to stop drinking once you've started
- You aren't able to do what's expected of you because of alcohol
- A friend or relative has expressed concern about your drinking.

EATING PROBLEMS

There are three main types of eating problem:

- Overeating
- Binge eating
- Undereating

Let's look at each of these in turn.

Overeating

More of us than ever before are overweight. Indeed, in 2009 a staggering 61 per cent of adults and 28 per cent of children in England were overweight or obese.

Our weight is the product of a combination of factors, from our genes and metabolism to our socio-economic group. Sometimes weight problems can be caused by physical factors, such as thyroid disease or some types of medications (for example, the contraceptive pill), but it's the fact that we eat so badly and exercise so rarely that's led to the recent rapid rise in the number of overweight people.

Most of us are just carrying a few extra pounds, but even so there are lots of good reasons to slim down. Losing just a little weight can make us feel happier, healthier and more energetic. And we'll also reduce the risk of developing serious illnesses such as cancer, heart disease, diabetes, strokes and arthritis.

Binge eating

In the mid 1970s doctors began to notice a new type of eating problem. The people affected – and they were almost all women – were prone to regular bouts of frenzied, uncontrolled eating. After these binges, they would attempt to compensate by vomiting, taking laxatives or other medications, dieting, fasting or exercising excessively. The behaviour seemed to be driven by a preoccupation with weight and appearance.

This problem is now known as *bulimia nervosa*, and it's very much at the severe end of the binge-eating spectrum. There are many people who don't meet the criteria for a diagnosis of bulimia but who still sometimes binge eat and vomit, while others binge eat but don't try to undo the effects of the food in some way afterwards.

It's estimated that at any time 5–10 per cent of women binge eat, with approximately 4.5 per cent of women between 18–24 suffering from bulimia.

Undereating

Most of us know what it's like to diet. The pressure on everyone, and especially women, to control our weight by eating less is arguably greater than ever. There are plenty of good reasons to maintain a healthy weight, but dieting isn't usually the answer, at least in the long term. Neither does it do much for our happiness, especially if – as usually happens – the weight just goes right back on when we stop dieting.

For a very small percentage of people – usually young women – the desire to be thin results in them consistently eating less than they need to maintain their normal body weight. And this behaviour continues even when they are seriously underweight. This is *anorexia nervosa*, and it can lead to serious health problems.

Like bulimia, anorexia is fuelled by the belief that what matters most is one's appearance – that self-esteem comes from slimness and self-control. About half of people with anorexia are also prone to bulimia-type behaviour.

SEXUAL PROBLEMS

Our culture is so saturated with sexual images and references that it's easy to believe there's something wrong with you if you're not constantly either having wonderfully fulfilling sex or thinking about it. But remember: whatever the state of your love life, it's only a problem if you – or your partner, if you're in a relationship – feel it is.

That said, when things aren't working out well in the bedroom life can seem pretty miserable. Sex, after all, is potentially a source of great pleasure, fulfilment and self-esteem and sexual problems can cause difficulties in relationships – which, as you'll remember from Chapter 8, are perhaps the most important source of happiness in our life.

Here's a brief summary of the most common sexual problems:

- **Absence of desire** – losing interest in sex. In any year, 40 per cent of women experience a loss of sexual desire that lasts at least a month.

- **Arousal problems** – though we want to have sex, our body doesn't respond accordingly. Over the course of a year, around 9 per cent of women will experience this problem for at least a month.

  In men, arousal problems are known as *erectile dysfunction*: the inability to develop or maintain an erection. Short-term difficulties are very common, but for around 15–20 per cent of men it's a persistent, significant problem. The risk increases with age.

- **Difficulties having an orgasm.** This is the most frequent reason why women seek sex therapy. Each year 14 per cent of women are unable to achieve an orgasm for at least a month. For 4 per cent, the problem lasts for six months or more.

- **Pain** – either during sex or even at the thought of it. This is generally a problem affecting women rather than men. Pain during intercourse is a persistent problem for around 12 per cent of women each year.

- **Premature ejaculation** is the most common sexual problem experienced by men. It's defined as consistently ejaculating sooner than you'd like. Around a third of men say that they ejaculate too quickly at least half the time.

HOW TO GET HELP

If you're struggling with any of the problems listed in this chapter, take heart: effective treatments are available for all of them.

One potentially valuable source of information and advice is self-help material – books, CDs and websites. There are many excellent self-help guides for all the problems we discuss in this chapter, and you can find some of them in the Further Reading section on pp. 157–8.

If you'd like to take things further, start by seeing your family doctor. Just chatting things over with your GP can be a huge help. If you think psychological therapy (also called 'psychotherapy' or 'talking therapy') might be useful, your doctor should be able to guide you through the options and make a referral. There are various types of psychotherapy but CBT is the one that's been proven to be most effective for these problems. Medication is also an option in some cases.

Incidentally, the UK's National Institute for Health and Clinical Excellence (NICE) produces guidelines on how best to treat psychological (as well as physical) problems. They're aimed primarily at health professionals, but there's no reason why you shouldn't consult them too. You'll also find summaries of the guidelines written specifically for the general public on their website: www.nice.org.uk.

And remember, emotional and psychological problems are normal. They're as much a part of life as any physical problem. Whatever you're going through, you can be certain that someone you know has had exactly the same problem at some stage of their lives. They came through it, and so will you.

CHAPTER 11

Becoming happier – and staying happier

Dedicate yourself to the good you deserve and desire for yourself. Give yourself peace of mind. You deserve to be happy. You deserve delight. HANNAH ARENDT (1906–75), GERMAN PHILOSOPHER

Psychologists have been debating the nature of happiness a great deal over recent years, and one of the central questions has been whether it's really possible to make a lasting change to our level of happiness.

The very good news – and the reason why we've written this book – is that research following people over time has shown it most definitely is possible. But in order to achieve those gains, it's best to have two key factors in place.

First of all, just wishing you were happier isn't enough (but you knew that already). Nor is simply changing your circumstances – for example, buying a new car, changing the way you dress, or moving to a new area. What matters is what you *do* and, more specifically, adopting the kind of targeted activities contained in this book.

The other key ingredient is one of approach. Make happiness a priority in your life; give it the prominence it deserves; build the activities into your daily routine. Achieving anything worthwhile takes effort, commitment and motivation – and becoming happier is no different. But you can do it. And it won't take very long before you begin to feel the benefits.

> *Make happiness a priority in your life;*
> *give it the prominence it deserves.*

The fact that you've made it this far in the book is proof that you're serious about wanting change. In the second part of this chapter, we'll suggest some techniques to help you keep going if your determination wavers. But let's start with a recap of the ground we've covered so far, and in particular the practical steps that will help increase your well-being.

> *Trust yourself. Create the kind of self that you will be happy to live with all your life. Make the most of yourself by fanning the tiny, inner sparks of possibility into flames of achievement.*
> GOLDA MEIR (1898–1978), ISRAELI PRIME MINISTER

BECOMING HAPPIER: A CHECKLIST

Here's the nutshell version of *You Can Be Happy*. You can use this summary to refresh your memory and as a checklist of activities to work through.

Key point:

Happiness is made up of four components:

- Pleasure.
- Meaning, that's to say connecting to something greater than yourself.
- Engagement, or losing yourself in an activity.
- Fewer negative emotions.

Our level of happiness is influenced by our life situation and our personality. Influenced, but not determined. Whatever your personal circumstances, you can become happier.

> *Whatever your personal circumstances,*
> *you can become happier.*

Activity:

- Measure your current level of happiness (p. 11).

Key point:

Just like any other skill, becoming happier requires effort, determination and motivation. To help you prepare, try the following exercises.

Activities:

- Weigh up the pros and cons of becoming happier (p. 16).
- Identify your role model, the inspirational figure whose story fills you with optimism, energy and joy (p. 18).
- Write your own tribute (p. 19).
- Develop a positive mindset (p. 21).

Key point:

You're more likely to be happy if you're eating healthily and sleeping well.

Activities:

- Book check-ups with your doctor and dentist (p. 27).

- See what you can do to improve your diet (p. 28).

- Tackle any sleep problems (p. 31).

Key point:

We can all improve how we feel by changing what we do. When it comes to boosting well-being, there are five key activities:

- Connect
- Be active
- Be curious
- Learn
- Give

Aim to add examples of each to your week. The activities listed below will help you.

Activities:

- Find activities that build on your strengths and values (p. 44).

- Reflect on activities you've enjoyed in the past (p. 47).

- Brainstorm enjoyable activities (p. 48).

- Keep an activities diary (p. 49).

- Set yourself goals (p. 51).

- Every day, do five things – no matter how small – that make you happy (p. 54).

Key point:

To be happier we must reduce the impact of negative emotions such as anxiety, sadness and anger.

Activities:

- Write about your emotions (p. 56).
- Learn to cope with worry (p. 57).
- Boost your problem-solving skills (p. 59).
- Be comfortable with your choices (p. 61).
- Tackle negative thoughts (p. 62).
- Develop your self-compassion (p. 64).
- Resist the temptation to compare yourself to others (p. 65).

Key point:

As well as calming our negative emotions, we need to increase our positive thoughts and feelings.

Activities:

- Ask yourself what's going right for you right now (p. 70).
- Savour the past, present and future (p. 70).
- Make gratitude a reflex (p. 72).
- Keep a diary of the positive things that happen to you (p. 74).
- Learn to exchange pessimism for optimism (p. 77).
- Use music and humour to boost your mood (p. 81).
- Smile! (p. 83)

Key point:

Learning how to relax your mind and body gives you a proven technique for increasing well-being. Make at least one of the following exercises part of your routine.

Activities:

- Progressive muscle relaxation (p. 86).
- Visualisation (p. 87).
- Mindfulness meditation (pp. 88–96).

Key point:

The stronger your relationships, the happier you're likely to be.

Activities:

- Build your social network (p. 98).
- Get to know the rules of friendship (p. 100).
- Express your gratitude (p. 102).
- Make praise a habit (p. 103).
- Remember what makes your friends special (p. 103).
- Be helpful (p. 104).
- Respond positively to good news (p. 104).
- Work to strengthen your relationship with your partner (pp. 108–16).

Key point:

We can all learn how to become happier at work. And considering how large a role work plays in most people's lives, that's a hugely important – and morale-boosting – message.

Activities:

- Strengthen your relationships at work (p. 120).
- Commit to your job (p. 121).
- Find meaning in your work (p. 123).
- Increase your level of control (p. 126).
- Develop your skills (p. 127).
- Look after yourself: don't let work dominate (p. 128).

Key point:

Sometimes unhappiness is a result of particular psychological problems. Among the most common are anxiety, depression, excessive anger, stress, difficulties with alcohol, and eating and sexual problems. If we understand what's troubling us, we're in a much better position to deal with it.

> *If we understand what's troubling us, we're in a much better position to deal with it.*

Activity:

Read through the descriptions of common problems and find out how to get treatment if you think it may be useful (pp. 133–44).

Staying happy

As you make the techniques in this book part of your life, you'll notice an upturn in your sense of well-being. There's no magic about this: put in the effort and you'll create the change you're looking for. As Woody Allen noted: 'Eighty per cent of success is showing up.' At regular intervals, revisit the happiness questionnaire on p. 11; you'll see just how far you've come.

But sticking with any life-changing programme can sometimes be tough. There are bound to be occasional days when you don't feel like going for a run, or meditating, or when negative thoughts get the better of you.

When a day like that occurs, don't let it get you down: it's normal. Remind yourself why you're working to increase your happiness. Remember just how much you've already achieved – and how much better you feel most of the time. Get back on the horse as soon as possible, and don't look back. What you've just experienced is a temporary diversion. It's not going to stop you getting where you want to be. Keep in mind the Buddhist saying: 'If we are facing in the right direction, all we have to do is keep on walking.'

To help you cope with those difficult days, draw up an *action plan*. Make a note of:

- The sorts of *stresses and problems* that are likely to lower your mood and sap your determination.

- The *early warning signs* that you're feeling down or lethargic.

- The *steps* you'll take to deal with these feelings.

Here's part of an action plan written by Laura, a 39-year-old nurse:

- *Stresses and problems*: Frantic days at work. When work is particularly busy and stressful, I feel more and more exhausted as the week goes on.

- *Early warning signs*: I try to meditate for ten minutes every day, but that's often the first thing to go when I'm tired. I might miss swimming on Thursday. I worry more. And I tend to eat less healthily – overdoing the chocolate and biscuits, for instance.

- *Steps to take:* Resist the temptation to stay up late and make sure I get plenty of sleep. Reward myself when I meditate – am more likely to do it if there's a treat at the end. Make sure I arrange for Jenny to pick me up for swimming; I won't want to let her down. Use worry periods. Don't keep sweet things in the house!

Keep your action plan somewhere accessible so you can find it when you need it.

> *When I thought I couldn't go on, I forced myself to keep going. My success is based on persistence, not luck.*
> ESTÉE LAUDER (1906–2004), US COSMETICS ENTREPRENEUR

You can reduce the chances of falling into a rut by varying your routine. If meditation, for example, isn't doing it for you at the moment, try yoga. If you've got into the habit of seeing the same friends in the same place on the same evening, shake things up. If jogging is starting to seem like a chore, try a new route, find a running mate, or perhaps try some other form of exercise.

> ❝ *You can reduce the chances of falling into a rut by varying your routine.* ❞

Remember also to make full use of your support network. If you feel your enthusiasm waning, share your feelings. Simply expressing your emotions to another person is usually a big help. Moreover, in return you're likely to receive sympathy, encouragement and support. And this is a time when you'll especially appreciate practical help, so don't be reticent about asking.

Over the past fifteen years happiness has received more attention from psychologists than ever before. The bottom line from all this research is simple and inspiring: we can all become happier.

There's no need to trust to chance. You can make it happen by following the scientifically proven techniques in this book. All it takes is a little belief, persistence and determination. We wish you well in your efforts.

> *Twenty years from now you will be more disappointed by the things that you didn't do than by the ones you did do. So throw off the bowlines. Sail away from the safe harbour. Catch the trade winds in your sails. Explore. Dream. Discover.* MARK TWAIN (1835–1910), US WRITER

Further reading

You Can Be Happy is all about the practical steps you can take to boost your happiness. We've kept the book as concise as possible so that you can focus on these key activities, but if you'd like to read more about the issues we cover, try the following titles:

Aaron Beck, *Love Is Never Enough: How Couples Can Overcome Misunderstandings, Resolve Conflicts, and Solve Relationship Problems Through Cognitive Therapy* (Harper, 1989)

David Burns, *Feeling Good: The New Mood Therapy* (Avon, 2000)

Gillian Butler, *Overcoming Social Anxiety and Shyness* (Robinson, 2009)

Colin Espie, *Overcoming Insomnia and Sleep Problems: A Self-help Guide Using Cognitive Behavioral Techniques* (Robinson, 2006)

Barbara Fredrickson, *Positivity: Groundbreaking Research to Release Your Inner Optimist and Thrive* (Oneworld, 2011)

Daniel Freeman and Jason Freeman, *Know Your Mind: Everyday Emotional and Psychological Problems and How to Overcome Them* (Rodale, 2009) – includes information on over fifty common problems.

HH the Dalai Lama and Howard Cutler, *The Art of Happiness at Work* (Mobius, 2005)

Jon Kabat-Zinn, *Wherever You Go, There You Are: Mindfulness Meditation for Everyday Life* (Piatkus, 2004)

Helen Kennerley, *Overcoming Anxiety* (Robinson, 2009)

Sonia Lyubomirsky, *The How of Happiness: A Practical Guide to Getting the Life You Want* (Piatkus, 2010)

Jessica Pryce-Jones, *Happiness at Work: Maximizing Your Psychological Capital for Success* (Wiley-Blackwell, 2010)

Mathieu Ricard, *Happiness: A Guide to Developing Life's Most Important Skill* (Little, Brown, 2007)

Martin Seligman, *Authentic Happiness: Using the New Positive Psychology to Realise Your Potential for Lasting Fulfilment* (Free Press, 2003)

Charlotte Style, *Brilliant Positive Psychology* (Prentice Hall, 2010)

Peter Warr and Guy Claperton, *The Joy of Work? Jobs, Happiness, and You* (Routledge, 2009)

Mark Williams and Danny Penman, *Mindfulness: A Practical Guide to Finding Peace in a Frantic World* (Piatkus, 2011)

Mark Williams, John Teasdale, Zindel Segal and Jon Kabat-Zinn, *The Mindful Way Through Depression: Freeing Yourself from Chronic Unhappiness* (Guilford, 2007)

Read On

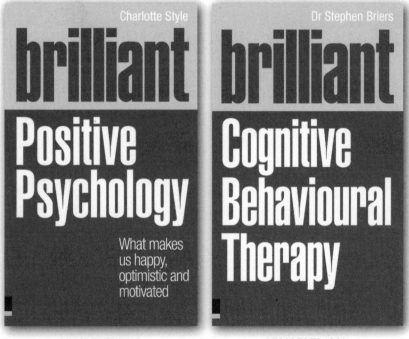

Available online and from all good book stores
www.pearson-books.com